The Evolution of HEALTH SERVICES RESEARCH

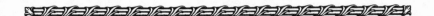

ODIN W. ANDERSON

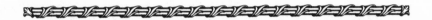

Foreword by James R. Greenley

The *Evolution of* HEALTH SERVICES RESEARCH

Personal Reflections on Applied Social Science

Jossey-Bass Publishers

San Francisco • Oxford • 1991

THE EVOLUTION OF HEALTH SERVICES RESEARCH
Personal Reflections on Applied Social Science
by Odin W. Anderson

Copyright © 1991 by: Jossey-Bass Inc., Publishers
350 Sansome Street
San Francisco, California 94104

&

Jossey-Bass Limited
Headington Hill Hall
Oxford OX3 0BW

Library of Congress Cataloging-in-Publication Data

Anderson, Odin W. (Odin Waldemar), date.
    The evolution of health services research : personal reflections
on applied social science / Odin W. Anderson.
        p.   cm.—(The Jossey-Bass health series)
    Includes bibliographical references.
    Includes index.
    ISBN 1-55542-340-X
    1. Medical care—Research—Government policy—United States—
History.   2. Medical care—Research—Social aspects—United States.
3. Social sciences—Research—United States—History.   4. Anderson,
Odin W. (Odin Waldemar), date.   5. Medical sociologists—
Wisconsin—Biography. I. Title. II. Series.
    [DNLM: 1. Health Services Research—history—United States.
2. Social Environment—history—United States.   3. Social Problems—
history—United States.   W 84.3 A548e]
RA395.A3A76   1991
362.1'072073—dc20
DNLM/DLC
for Library of Congress   90-15644
                                                                      CIP

Manufactured in the United States of America

The paper in this book meets the guidelines for
permanence and durability of the Committee on
Production Guidelines for Book Longevity of the
Council on Library Resources.

JACKET DESIGN BY WILLI BAUM
FIRST EDITION

Code 9143

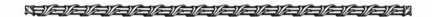

The Jossey-Bass Health Series

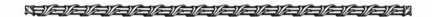

*This book is dedicated to Nathan Sinai (1894–1974),
professor of public health, University of Michigan.
From 1942 to 1949, he inducted me into health services
research and teaching, which was then a new field,
and provided the springboard for the rest of my
professional life.*

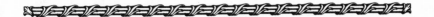

Contents

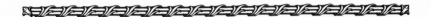

Foreword

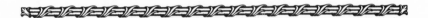

In this fine book by Odin Anderson, the ancient advice "Know thyself" is given to those whose work bridges social science and public policy. The reader will no doubt find, as I did, that the book helps him or her follow this advice by aiding self-reflection and understanding. This is a book likely to engage the reader personally, in a way that treatises on these topics rarely, if ever, do.

The book begins with a discussion of turn-of-the-century social reformers and social scientists such as Edward A. Ross, John L. Gillin, and William F. Ogburn. These leaders believed that social research would contribute to the amelioration of social problems. They launched generations of scholars, including the author of this book, into social research, which was conceived of as a tool in the social engineering of society. These reformers envisioned the good society in terms of a liberal-democratic tradition. They failed to recognize the part their values played in shaping their vision but took their view of the good society as self-evident.

Later critics of these early social reformers pointed out that the unstated values and hidden assumptions embedded in the work of these "social engineers." In the decades following World War II, this critical perspective was widely held, and many social scientists abandoned efforts to find solutions to social problems through social research. From this critical perspective, all social research was value-laden. If social problems were the result of value conflicts, then social scientists were no better than politicians. In his sociohistorical conceptualization, Anderson performs the useful and engaging task of getting me (and, I suspect, most readers) to see their lives and work in the context of the "social engineering" and "social-sciences-as-politics" perspectives.

The book proceeds with a discussion of four major research projects, including the Coleman Report and the Moynihan Report. The discussion highlights the interest groups that form the political context in which research takes place. Issues are brought out, in various ways, in descriptions of the lives and work of eighteen prominent social scientists. Many but not all of them have worked in the health services areas. Some are Anderson's contemporaries, and others belong to later generations of researchers. Their lives and work embody the issues, dilemmas, and problems encountered by predominantly reform-oriented researchers of social problems. These issues and problems include academic freedom, working with the press, pressures from funding sources, dealing with unpopular results, and others.

This subject is plumbed more elaborately and poignantly in the author's detailed account of his own life and career. In his discussion of his boyhood, his university education, his work in New York for the Health Information Foundation, his research and teaching at the University of Chicago, and his subsequent move to the University of Wisconsin, Anderson presents numerous telling examples of his own social policy–oriented research.

The extensive autobiographical data and details constitute a vibrant and stimulating strength of the book. Readers can begin to understand Anderson's research because they begin to understand the man. We learn that Odin Anderson was orphaned at the age of two and was brought up as a foster child in a household of his older aunts and uncles and his paternal grandmother, "in the family but not of it." This was a rural Norwegian-American family on the fringes of a town dominated by the Anglo elite. His experiences gave him the outsider's perspective on social phenomena that is so common to social scientists. These personal stories and anecdotes weave a tapestry against which his reactions to the challenges and pressures presented by funding sources and publishers can be understood. By giving these details about his own life, the author challenges and stimulates readers to recall similar key events and formative stages in their lives and relate them to their experiences with social research.

Anderson is one of only a handful of eminent, influential, productive scholars who could have written a book like this one. He started out on a dairy farm in rural Wisconsin and went on to study sociology at the University of Wisconsin and the University of Michigan, where he received his Ph.D. degree. He was a pioneer in the health services research field before it was known as such. He has been a prolific author and researcher, tackling the central problems of the time, such as financing or equity in access to health care. Widely traveled and respected as an international scholar of health services, he has the respect of policymakers and researchers in many countries beyond our own. He has trained a very large number of health services researchers and, in this way, has put his mark on the field.

This book suggests that several different contexts form policy-oriented social research and reactions to it. One context is the unique life experiences of the participants, dealt with so well in this book. Also thoroughly presented, within the autobiographical framework, are the organizational contexts, the professional contexts, and the broader historical and political contexts. Anderson makes clear that the Health Information Foundation and the University of Chicago's Graduate School of Business, where he worked, were organizational contexts that could either facilitate or preclude research. For example, the professional context limited the research and results that colleagues would take seriously; results or interpretations that seemed inconsistent with the predominantly liberal professional bias were commonly ignored, attacked, or rejected. The historical and political contexts, for instance, were evident in the antagonism directed toward Anderson's research on health maintenance organizations by physicians and private insurance companies. The strength and vehemence of these professional and organizational interests created a stressful research environment for Anderson. At one point, he was summarily thrown out of a meeting of the Group Health Association. He had to live with the possibility that some powerful group, conservative or liberal, would take offense at his work and successfully move to cut off his research funding or get him fired. It was risky to publicize research results. At times, he and his research were attacked by the American Medical Association, from the right, and simultaneously by the more liberal Group Health Association. As Anderson argues, survival as an effective policy researcher in such an environment is more likely when the researcher understands these conflicting forces and contexts. Unlike some of the other researchers whose lives and work are described in this book, Anderson not only survived these stressful organizational and professional contexts but also thrived, with objectivity and integrity.

The author challenges us to be aware of these contexts and to know the organizations, professionals, and interest groups better than they know themselves. By becoming an insider to their ways, the researcher can avoid being co-opted or dominated by them. Nevertheless, researchers must understand where their own goals and values are in relation to these other landscapes—hence the appeal to self-knowledge.

The discussion of these contexts also brings in the involvement of a wide range of people whose lives and work are connected to social research. These include researchers, governmental and private research funders, professional health and other administrators (such as those in the pharmaceutical industry), physicians, editors, publishers, reporters and newspeople, politicians, and citizen advocates for policy positions. Thus, many types of people will see themselves in this book and will be stimulated and intellectually challenged by reading it.

February 1991

James R. Greenley
Professor of Sociology and Psychiatry
University of Wisconsin–Madison

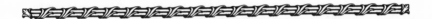

Preface

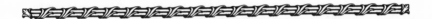

Health services research has attained the status of a truly interdisciplinary area. Its beginnings were as early as 1928–1933, when the Committee on the Costs of Medical Care (CCMC), funded by several philanthropic foundations, was in operation. The purpose of CCMC in those days was to find out, through a nationwide household survey, what Americans were paying for the health services they used and what Americans' patterns of sickness were. The survey was meant to establish a beginning benchmark on which to base rational public policy for private and public programming of American health services. In 1935–1936, this survey was followed by a massive survey of illnesses in the American population, conducted by the U.S. Public Health Service. I am an academic descendant of that first CCMC survey. In 1942, at the University of Michigan's School of Public Health, I was hired by Professor Nathan Sinai, one of three researchers who conducted the survey, to be his assistant and help him continue opening up the field of health services research.

This book is about the general development of health services research. It draws on the careers of some twenty colleagues, discussing their experiences in an area of research that was very controversial at first. It also draws on research in civil liberties and race relations and on experience within the Catholic Church. The research was controversial because it touched the sensitivities of interest groups (hospitals, the medical profession and allied health professions, insurance companies, employers and government as sources of funding, and the general public); in my own experience, from 1942 to the present, I have learned, as others also have done, to pick my way through a political minefield.

This book does not deal with technical or methodological problems in health services research. Rather, its purpose is to describe reciprocal relationships within the political environment of research, as well as researchers' experiences with those relationships. In courses on social research methodology, rarely is any attention paid to the political context of the research; yet it is an important variable that can motivate researchers who are aware of it to gain access to information and agencies and to anticipate interest groups' reactions to research findings. Since researchers—particularly those working on applied research related to public policy—are social animals and therefore are implicated in the problems they study, the book concludes with some guidelines for applied research. Throughout the book, I have used the stages of my own research career to reflect on the reciprocal relationships discussed here.

Overview of the Contents

The introductory chapter covers my intellectual and political heritage. My social and political environment in rural Wisconsin was shaped during the height of the Progressive era in Wisconsin politics. At the University of Wisconsin–Madison in the thirties, this heritage was intellectually enforced by the political atmosphere on the campus, the faculty I encountered, and like-minded students. This was the heady period of Roosevelt New Deal liberalism, which has been attenuated but continues to be subliminal in the social and political soul-searching of American politics. This changing and complex environment was the context within which my research career developed.

Chapter Two deals with the issue of "solving" social problems with social research. Applied social research for social problem solving gained great momentum during the presidency of Lyndon B. Johnson in his War on Poverty. In this chapter, I present four social research projects from the early sixties to the late seventies selected because of the intense attention they received from interest groups in American society at that time. These projects revealed that social research on problems touching interested parties, such as the causes of poverty among both whites and blacks, but particularly among blacks, was inevitably biased. The projects raised a storm of debate as to the research methodology and interpretation of results. Three of the projects were related to poverty and education, and the fourth dealt with American military intervention in South American countries to discourage Communist takeovers.

Chapter Three is on working in applied social research. It describes a selective sample of people and projects I encountered in this area. I selected eighteen research projects, mostly in the health field, except for one affiliated with a poverty research institute and another on the problem of recruiting priests in the Catholic Church. I know all the researchers personally. These researchers encountered a range of problems with access to data sources, relationships with agencies that were research subjects, publication of controversial results, and sources of funding. Otherwise the researchers were generally successful in completing and publishing their results.

In Chapter Four I describe my early formative social environment, covering the period from 1914 to 1942. In this chapter, I set forth in detail the personal circumstances that shaped my philosophy of life and my way of dealing with the world as revealed in my research career. A very important factor was my becoming an orphan at the age of two and being raised by my father's mother and siblings on a dairy farm in western Wisconsin. The rural area in which I grew up was almost exclusively Norwegian, a cultural enclave, and I became bilingual and bicultural. Suffice it to say that I became an observer whose interest turned to journalism and sociology and eventually to medical sociology. In 1942 I had my first job as research assistant to a professor of public health at the University of Michigan. This appointment started my continuous career in the health services field.

Chapter Five describes the ten years, from 1942 to 1952, that laid the basis for my career. Between 1942 and 1949 I received my Ph.D. degree in sociology at the University of Michigan and began to establish a teaching and research career in the School of Public Health there. I was due for a tenure-track position at the School of Public Health but resigned to accept a tenure-track associate professorship in the Faculty of Medicine, University of Western Ontario, Canada. In the Faculty of Medicine I moved into study and research in epidemiology, particularly the emerging area of social epidemiology. I also began to work in the utilization of physicians' services in a nearby medical insurance plan.

Chapter Six recounts my years as research director of the Health Information Foundation, spanning the period from 1952 to 1962. This research agency was founded by the drug, pharmaceutical, and chemical industries in 1950 to provide information and data for public policy formulation in the United States. It was a nonprofit, tax-exempt educational and research agency set up as a public service by the industries. Early in 1952 I was offered the position of research director; my task was to develop a research program. The foundation became a spectacular success through the research programs I developed and financed through my sponsors. I directed and sponsored research in the health services that had direct policy implications and established research on cross-national comparisons of the operation of health services delivery systems and health insurance. By 1960 the University of Chicago invited us to make the foundation a complement to its graduate program in hospital administration. We then entered a new era for the foundation.

Chapter Seven continues the story of my work at the Health Information Foundation in its University of Chicago phase, from 1962 to 1980. The move to the University of Chicago in 1962 gave the foundation and staff a stable operating base and a new name, the Center for Health Administration Studies. We floated many research projects during this time funded from various sources, but particularly from the National Center for Health Services Research in the Department of Health, Education, and Welfare, which awarded us two programmatic grants for seven years. I continued and developed my cross-national comparisons research and succeeded the director of the center when he retired in 1970. After my own retirement in 1980, I continued part-time until 1990. During that same period I had a half-time professorial appointment in the Department of Sociology at the University of Wisconsin–Madison, which I still hold. I was also appointed to the faculty of the Program in Health Services Management at the University of Wisconsin.

Occupying teaching and research positions at two major universities at the same time was a fascinating experience, which is described in Chapter Eight. One major difference between the two universities was that the University of Wisconsin was a publicly sponsored university whereas the University of Chicago was a private university. At Wisconsin I was constantly conscious of the state legislature and its influence. At Chicago I felt the university to be almost completely free of such influence. During that decade I published four books and several articles. They represent a research momentum facilitated by my Chicago position beginning in 1962 and continued at Wisconsin.

In Chapter Nine I present lessons for applied social science researchers gleaned from my own experience. The three major lessons, among many others listed in this chapter, are:

1. Applied research means studying a particular institution, such as a hospital, or a specific problem, such as access to health services. To be of help to the field, the applied social science researcher needs to be even more knowledgeable about the institution or problem than the person who works within the system.
2. Vested interests are involved in accepting or rejecting results of applied research. The first attack in case of rejection is on the methodology. Hence, applied social science researchers should use only well-tested methodology. Experimenting with methodology makes them too vulnerable.
3. Researchers should know themselves thoroughly so as to recognize personal biases and predilections. Health services researchers become marginal to the main disciplines and must be able to operate between sectors and have no particular identification with any of them.

Chapter Ten contains a self-assessment of my key contributions to health services research. I believe my key contribution has been both a macroanalysis of health services delivery systems in the United States and cross-national comparisons. I have tried to show which factors are constantly problematic in the health services, such as the physician-patient relationship and the interface between need/demand and the service institution. And I have tried to show which problems are quite solvable once a consensus is reached, such as legislating universal health insurance to eliminate the financial cost of services at time of service. Access issues and financial issues are always problematic; the solution to the problem of getting universal health insurance is quite mechanical given the political will.

Acknowledgments

The Graduate School of the University of Wisconsin–Madison provided seed money to help me develop this book. It enabled me to engage Mark Solovey, a graduate student in history and science, to make a thorough search of the literature on social research as it is related to public policy. I wish to mention the many colleagues whose enthusiasm for this book sustained my belief in its potential contribution to what could be called the sociology of social research and public policy. I also wish to thank the University of Wisconsin–Madison in general, and the Department of Sociology in particular, for providing me, by their very nature and style, with a congenial setting and atmosphere for working on this book. Finally, I wish to thank Sandra Ramer, assisted by Toni Schulze, for her stellar typing and for her patience and ability in reading my handwriting; this late in my life, I have not bothered to master the word processor and its associated technology.

Madison, Wisconsin   Odin W. Anderson
February 1991

The Author

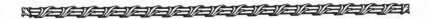

Odin W. Anderson is professor of sociology at the University of Wisconsin-Madison. He is also professor emeritus of sociology, University of Chicago. He received his B.A. and M.A. degrees (1937 and 1938, respectively) from the University of Wisconsin-Madison in sociology, his B.A. degree (1940) from the University of Michigan in library science, and his Ph.D. degree (1948) from the University of Michigan in sociology. He holds honorary degrees from the Faculty of Medicine, University of Uppsala, Sweden (1977), and the College of Osteopathic Medicine, Chicago (1979).

Anderson's main research has been in the macro aspects of health services delivery in the United States and cross-nationally. He was awarded the title of Distinguished Medical Sociologist by the Section on Medical Sociology, American Sociological Association (1980), and the title of Distinguished Health Services Researcher by the Association of Health Services Research (1985). His publications include *Family Medical Costs and Voluntary Health Insurance: A Nationwide Survey* (1956, with J. J. Feldman), *Health Services in the United States: A Growth Enterprise Since 1875* (1985), and *The Health Services Continuum in Democratic States: An Inquiry into Solvable Problems* (1989).

The Evolution of HEALTH SERVICES RESEARCH

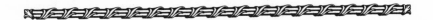

1

Introduction:
My Intellectual
and Political Heritage

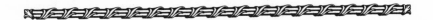

A section on the sociology of medicine was established within the American Sociological Association in 1960. It quickly became one of the largest sections. A decade or so before, a few sociologists had begun to take an interest in medical sociology (although that term had not yet been coined). Research in health services later expanded beyond sociology. Not long after that, economists, political scientists, and operations researchers became engaged in increasing numbers, as the health services became the third-largest industry in the country (measured by total expenditures, in comparison with other industries). Philanthropic foundations—and, soon afterward, the federal government—became interested in funding research by the several disciplines after World War II, as problems in health services delivery began to evoke greater and greater private and public political interest. One consequence of this interest has been the creation of a very large cadre of health services researchers from the various disciplines.

My own career has spanned the entire period of this development, and I have been fortunate enough to be at the right place at the right time, with respect to research positions as well as funding sources. This book relates my career to the economic and political contexts of health services and to the health services research that evolved in those contexts. I have tried to show how my life history, the environment conditioning my political philosophy, and my personal characteristics have meshed; as this book will show, one's choice of research projects and the evolution of health

1

services delivery systems flow from values, rather than from facts, since facts may either support or cast doubt on the practicality of values. I have divided my career into five stages.

1. From 1932 to 1938, I was a student at the University of Wisconsin–Madison, in the depths of the Great Depression and immediately before World War II. I had intended to become a journalist but eventually became a sociologist. I was a child of the Progressive period in Wisconsin and national politics. My professors were strongly oriented toward public policy because of the Depression, and I was greatly influenced to study policy problems, rather than theoretical problems. Health services research had barely started.

2. In 1938, with a master's degree in sociology from Wisconsin, I went to the University of Michigan. I wanted to become a college librarian. After earning a B.A. in library science, however, I returned to sociology for a Ph.D. (I had been told that a Ph.D. would be helpful in becoming the director of a university library). The combination of these two backgrounds resulted in my becoming a research assistant to Professor Nathan Sinai and helping him develop a research program in medical care at the School of Public Health (see Chapter Five). He also wished to establish a health services research library. I became the first sociologist to work in a school of public health, where I remained from 1942 to 1949. I was also establishing a reputation in health services research. I received my Ph.D. in sociology in 1948.

3. In 1949, I accepted an offer to become an associate professor of the social aspects of medicine at the Faculty of Medicine, University of Western Ontario. While there, from 1949 to 1952, I worked mainly in social epidemiology, rather than in health services as such. I had become the first full-time academic sociologist in a medical school. During that time, I published some work on morbidity and mortality patterns as they were related to social variables.

4. My big break came in 1952 (although I was not sure it would be a break). The drug, pharmaceutical, and chemical industries had established the Health Information Foundation in New

York City, to conduct objective research in the health services and provide facts for the rational formulation of public policy (rather than brickbats for purveyors of misinformation). I became the research director and, as it turned out, was given virtual control of an annual budget of $400,000, for research with my own staff and for grants to researchers in universities. We made three nationwide household surveys (of health services use, expenditures, attitudes, and so on). These established us in the field and became a source of information for all interested groups. I also began cross-national research in 1958, by going to Sweden and the United Kingdom, where I returned annually for the next thirty years. I was research director for ten years; then there was a change of board members, and a feeling developed that the three industries had contributed enough. The upshot was that the Graduate School of Business at the University of Chicago invited the foundation and its staff to take over the graduate program in hospital administration and conduct a ready-to-go research program already developed in New York. In the summer of 1962, we moved to the University of Chicago, taking a reserve fund of $1 million with us. The foundation was renamed the Center for Health Administration Studies. I continued as research director and, in addition, became a professor in the Graduate School of Business and in the Department of Sociology. We flourished with research funds from philanthropic foundations and from the federal government. My cross-national research also flourished. We became a model and reference point for health services research. From all reports, we had great influence on the field.

5. In 1980, I reached compulsory retirement age and was preparing to move to Madison, Wisconsin, to retire. When my intentions became known at the University of Wisconsin, its Department of Sociology offered me a half-time professorship, to carry on teaching and research. The University of Chicago also hired me half-time, and I taught at both universities for ten years, until 1990. During that time, I conducted a health-maintenance organization (HMO) study in Minneapolis–St. Paul and Chicago, wrote a book on health services of seven countries, and wrote a history of the development of American health services

since 1875; all were published. I plan now to continue at the University of Wisconsin–Madison indefinitely, according to my continued competence and interests.

My approach to this book is quite straightforward. I use both primary and secondary sources. The secondary resources are books and articles by social scientists whom I regard as colleagues and who have pondered and had experience with policy-oriented research, in terms of both theory and application. I use these sources to show the sociopolitical and academic contexts in which they were written, and which are also pertinent to my career. As for the primary sources, I conducted correspondence and had face-to-face or telephone interviews with some twenty social scientists who have been or are now engaged in policy-oriented research, and I asked them about their experience.

A major source of the material presented as my personal experience is my recollections of my research career, taken from memory and from minutes, correspondence, and documents of the Health Information Foundation. I also draw on correspondence and documents from the Center for Health Administration Studies at the University of Chicago, from 1962 to 1990.

This, then, is a case study of a single research career in applied social science. It includes vignettes from other social scientists, and these vignettes are placed in social, political, and academic contexts, in relation to emerging and current issues in health services. I do not consider myself a research methodologist, in the sense of using rigid designs and sophisticated quantitative analysis, although I have borrowed methodologies and have had excellent methodological collaborators. Nor have I made any direct attempts to contribute to social theory: any theoretical concepts that may appear in my writing are those that I have absorbed from wide reading in history, political science, economics, and sociology (I am voraciously eclectic). What I do claim, from many years of first-hand exposure as an academician and researcher, is a very deep absorption in the health services as a social system. I have cultivated relationships with a whole range of front-line people in health services administration, medical care, public health, health insurance, and politics. I have worked at becoming acquainted with the issues politically, economically, and administratively. I have always been a macroanalyst; microanalysis is not congenial to my style of viewing the world, either scientifically or personally. In an age of specialization, I aspired to be a macroanalyst of the health services and their ramifications. Even here, however, I am sure that I am an endangered species. I see specialization all around me—a necessary aspect of scientific evolution, although it has its costs (such as inability to see the whole—fiddle with one sector of the health services delivery system, even a small one, and a ripple runs through the whole system, and another problem pops up somewhere else).

My Heritage

To show the relationship between my research career and the intellectual and political heritage that shaped my views and my research, I will give a brief background on the roots of that heritage in my upbringing and education. Too often, I believe, social researchers are only dimly aware of the sources of their values and take them as given. In developing my social research strategy, as related to public policy, I felt a need to bring the roots of my own values to the surface.

For a hundred and fifty years or so (since the time of August Comte in France, Eilert Sundt in Norway, and Lester Ward in the United States, to mention three early and well-known social scientists), social scientists have been active in propounding their particular concepts of the good society. Such concepts have been formulated within social and political theories, ranging from laissez-faire capitalism to communism, from technocracy to interest-group political processes. These pioneers were unabashed in stating their beliefs about what constituted the good society, and they did not worry about whether their views were value-free. In fact, they took their views as given, in the nature of things. This state of affairs in the social sciences held sway with little question until World War II. In the late 1930s, there were some glimmers of criticism regarding the simplistic nature of the theory of social problems and how to solve them. Shortly thereafter in the United States, sociologists began to theorize about how social problems came to be defined as problems and accompanied by theories of social change and of possibilities for directed change. Debates over value-neutral and value-loaded social science research began in 1945, after World War II had ended.

So much for the general aspects of my heritage. More directly, I was taught by those in social sciences and in the humanities who had one foot in the nineteenth century and the other in the twentieth. My college years (1932–1938) at the University of Wisconsin–Madison were spent in the presence of professors whose education and outlook were shaped by the latter nineteenth century's and the early twentieth century's faith in science, reason, and education as gateways to the good society. Those scholars' social and political values were a given; they embodied what became known as the Progressive era (from roughly 1880 to the 1930s or so). Progress was everywhere: more education; rising production and standards of living; eradication of the major disease scourges of humankind; extension of voting rights to all adult men, regardless of social status, and, later, to women; improved and faster land transportation; railroads and the automobile. World War I (1914–1918) chastened the adult generation of that time with respect to those firmly held progressive values; the carnage in Europe was a shock. Nevertheless, my American mentors regained their optimism; and their students, my contemporaries, maintained their confidence (as I also did), even during the Great Depression, that human progress was only temporarily blunted.

I was born in 1914, in Minneapolis, to rising middle-class parents. My father had a staff job as a freight salesman in the railroad business, which was peaking by 1914. He had grown up on a dairy farm. In a family of fourteen brothers and sisters, he was the second oldest. He attended high school in a small Wisconsin town and business college in Minneapolis. He was the son of Norwegian immigrants. My mother, too, was born to Norwegian immigrants, in Iowa. She went to Minneapolis and became a seamstress. There she met my father. In 1916, she contracted pulmonary tuberculosis and was placed in a sanitarium to die. I was taken to my father's farm home and cared for by my father's sister, then twenty-two years old; my father, awaiting my mother's death, was going to rearrange his life and take me back. But three weeks after my mother died, in 1917, my father contracted erysipelas and also died. I simply remained on the farm and grew up with my father's extended family in western Wisconsin.

In this family of my father's ten siblings (my uncles and aunts) and my grandmother, I was five years younger than the youngest child, a seven-year-old girl. I was in the family but not of it. My father left a modest but significant legacy, which made me college-bound early on. I believe that my experience of being in but not of this very supportive family made me into an observer and, later, led to my interest in journalism and sociology.

We lived in a densely populated township of dour Lutheran Norwegian immigrants and their descendants. We were bilingual— we spoke Norwegian at home and with neighbors, and English at school and in business. We had a sense of "them" (non-Norwegians) and "us" (Norwegians), although the relationships were friendly and symbiotic. These influences, I believe, trained me to be a marginal actor, a role that I feel has characterized my professional life. My Lutheran training, compounded by the unpredictability of the weather and its consequences for farmers, imprinted on me an essentially tragic view of life. I became a Unitarian in college, but the Lutheran heritage stays on, minus the theology.

The farmers in the area were ardent Progressives. As I was growing up, I too became ardently Progressive, an orientation I retained through the founding of the New Deal, during the Depression of the 1930s. I was then an undergraduate at the University of Wisconsin–Madison and entered into the politically liberal atmosphere of that school. After "bumming around" academically, so to speak, I finally found an outlet in sociology and institutional economics. The social science faculty were quite strongly oriented toward applied social science and policy, and I thrived in that atmosphere. Ever since, I have been an applied research sociologist.

Before the "Value-Free" Issue

At the turn of the twentieth century, and up to 1940 or so, leaders in economics and sociology seemed to have no qualms about their role as social scientists and their role as advocates of what they regarded as the good and just society. They used systematic data collection to support their advocacy, particularly in Wisconsin, where it seemed natural to use government (together with private enterprise, with government as the instrument and catalyst) to improve the lot of the working-class population and the farmers, to keep children out of factories and put them in school, and to fight alcoholism and crime. This social philosophy went against the grain of big industry and business, whose leaders subscribed to the laissez-faire philosophy and embodied, in crude form, Darwin's theory of the survival of the fittest.

How university-based scholars like Richard T. Ely, John R. Commons, and Edward Alsworth Ross survived and even flourished in this type of political and economic atmosphere is a story in itself. Here, we must examine their environment briefly, as a prelude to our discussion of the emergence of applied social research (particularly applied to politically sensitive social problems). Fortunately, there are very good secondary sources that help to provide a background (see Hofstadter and Metzger, 1955; Curti and Carstenson, 1949).

As Hofstadter and Metzger point out, even the universities of the Middle Ages enjoyed a certain modicum of freedom in that they were closely integrated with the monarchy and the church: "If the universities were spiritual centers, they were scarcely less important as agencies of practical life, whose work was as relevant to the ecclesiastical and political life of the thirteenth and fourteenth centuries as the modern university is to the scientific and industrial life of our time" (Hofstadter and Metzger, 1955, p. 6).

From the modern perspective, it is difficult to conceive of academic freedom as existing in the universities of the Middle Ages; but Hofstadter and Metzger point out the unique need for universities to be free (within ideological bounds) because society needed them, just as society needs them now (still within broad ideological bounds, short of violent revolution). The methodology of the scholastics of that time was dialectic: it fed the masters' need for a clash of mind against mind. Later, the methodology became empirical— physical and biological research, which led to naturalistic views of the cosmos and of biology and undermined orthodox religious doctrines. Still later, social scientists emerged, during the latter nineteenth and early twentieth centuries, and they began to challenge economic and political doctrines. By this time, civil and academic freedom from religious orthodoxy had been largely attained, and the churches were on the defensive.

The new battleground was the freedom of economists and sociologists to conduct empirical research on economic and social problems, which, by definition, were enmeshed in the conservative economic and political ideology of the day. Among economists and sociologists there was, however, a split concerning the role of the state in the daily lives of the people, beyond ensuring order through the courts and the police and ensuring the sanctity of voluntary contracts and the sovereignty of the people (through periodic elections to "turn the rascals out"). A minority of economists devoted themselves to institutional economics, a melding of sociology, economics, and political science; the majority embraced both the laissez-faire market economy and the doctrine of limited interference by the state. By contrast, the great majority of sociologists, with their concepts of social organization and social systems, supported state intervention: they regarded the state as an organic part of society, rather than as another interest group divorced from society. In fact, it seems that sociologists did not think in terms of the economy at all, or of what it would cost to implement their recommendations, and this is still largely true. Important exceptions, like Herbert Spencer in England and William Graham Sumner in the United States, espoused a concept of society that resembled the concept of the laissez-faire economists. The political and economic milieu of Wisconsin, and of the upper Midwest generally, found expression at the University of Wisconsin–Madison. Through its university, Wisconsin became an academic leader in the Progressive era, from the turn of the century into the 1930s, particularly in the social sciences. The sociologists at the University of Chicago were cast in somewhat the same mold, but they lacked the congenial political atmosphere of Wisconsin.

The country, of course, was going through a tremendous economic transformation, from an agricultural to an industrial society. Cities, growing rapidly, were giving rise to slums and terrible working conditions in mines and factories, to abject poverty, to crimes against life and property, to low wages, to unhealthful working conditions, and to toil from early in the morning to late at night. Nevertheless, a productive economy created, in time, enough of a surplus to raise wages and establish social insurance programs. No one was to blame for these conditions; they were systemic. The feverish pace of development at this time is captured by the American historian Daniel Boorstin, who wrote many years later, "The years after the Civil War when the continent was only partly explored were the halcyon days of the Go-Getters. They went in search of what others had never imagined was there to get. The Go-Getters made something out of nothing. They brought meat out of the desert, found oil in the rocks and brought light to millions. They discovered new resources, and where there seemed none to be discovered, they invented new ways of profiting from others who were trying to invent and to discover" (Boorstin, 1973, p. 3). There was a vast continent to conquer in a short time; and, very important, there was a large reservoir of entrepreneurial talent available and ready to exploit the enormous influx of immigrant labor from all over the world.

The leaders of the Wisconsin School, as it was called, were originally economists. When they saw the results of unbridled capitalism, they became sociologists, as well as continuing to be economists who had great interest in the political process. These leaders were Richard T. Ely, appointed to the faculty in 1982 and tasked with heading a new school of economics, political science, and history; John R. Commons, appointed by Ely in 1904 to teach economics; and Edward Alsworth Ross, whom Ely hired in 1906 to teach sociology (Ely, 1938). They became known as institutional economists (although Ross continued to regard himself as a sociologist). They were not opposed to capitalism, as such; they recognized the need for self-interest incentives based on profit. They did, however, work toward correcting and mitigating the excesses of exploitive capitalism by supporting labor unions as a countervailing force to the entrepreneurs, regulating working conditions and hours, and delineating the differences between services and products (like public utilities) that do not lend themselves to competition and those (like automobile manufacturing) that do lend themselves to competition. They wanted to prevent monopolies and foster competition through regulation.

All three men received part of their training in German universities of the latter nineteenth century. At these universities, professors in the social sciences regarded society as an organic whole that could be made orderly and productive through the blending of private enterprise and state intervention (although this would be the intervention of a paternalistic state inherited from the Middle Ages). By the late 1800s, Germany already had labor unions, social insurance, factory laws, and so on—all products of state intervention. Such influences notwithstanding, these American students recognized the uniqueness of the American experience and believed deeply in the capacity of the American democratic and political process to improve society.

This improvement would be brought about through systematic social research on the problems at hand. Many times, such research led to conflict with the industrial and business powers because the recommendations for reforming society fostered labor unions, a minimum wage, and workers' compensation, which all, of course, impinged on profit margins and entrepreneurial freedom. Nevertheless, the increasingly productive economy was eventually able to finance these ameliorative measures in one way or another.

All three men were social science eclectics. Ely wrote that, among economists at that time, "there was a striving for righteousness and perhaps here and there might have been one who felt a certain kinship to the old Hebrew prophets" (Ely, 1938, p. 143). Ross expressed the same view in his autobiography (Ross, 1936). Commons (1964, p. 143) wrote, "I was trying to save capitalism by making it good." In 1912, Ross brought John L. Gillin to the school, and Gillin began to teach courses in sociology. He had been a minister in an evangelical denomination and, fired by the "social gospel" doctrine of the time, carried his mission into sociology. His early courses, while they cannot be regarded as theoretical sociology, did describe the major social problems of the day and suggest solutions (the production of systematic data was expected to lead to quite self-evident solutions in an enlightened political democracy).

Ross (1924) produced a theory of society in his *Social Control*, which thrust him into leadership in American sociology. Very important, however, is the fact that his book was contemporaneous with the Progressive era; Weinberg (1972, p. 89) observes that the book enormously enhanced Ross's reputation among Progressive reformers. "The popularity of Ross's work rested on several counts: the timeliness of its appearance, the clarity with which Ross delineated the implications of America's transformation from a rural-commercial economy to an industrial-urban order, the enormous scholarship he brought to bear on his major thesis, and the appealing quality of the solutions he proposed to the problems confronting people at the turn of the century. Praise naturally came from his colleagues in sociology already familiar with his work, and from Progressive-minded editors, teachers, ministers, social workers and even literate politicians."

Still, Ely and Ross, even though they were seated in a university that was becoming a leader in propounding academic freedom for scholars, had to be sensitive to the possibility of attack from the enormous economically and politically conservative forces in the country. The natural and physical scientists had few problems in this respect, as far as the churches were concerned by this time, but the academic freedom of social scientists was being tested. Ross had left Stanford University for the University of Nebraska under pressure, applied because of his views on the importation of cheap Chinese labor by industrialists (he said the practice depressed the wages of American workers), his support of labor unions, and his attacks on railroads' monopolies. Stanford University was supported in large part by the railroad tycoon Leland Stanford. It was because of his reformative views that Ross was eventually invited to the University of Wisconsin.

Ely came under attack by big business in 1894, for the usual Progressive reforms he espoused, but he was supported by the University of Wisconsin's administration. In fact, a "trial," as reported by Curti and Carstenson (1949), was held to learn more about Ely's views. Ross came under attack in 1910, for inviting the self-styled anarchist Emma Goldman to speak to his class about her views, with which Ross disagreed. Ross supported free speech, but the university's president felt that Ross had made a serious mistake in judgment. Still, at a meeting of the board of regents on March 2, 1910, the president successfully thwarted the movement to oust Ross. He told the board that to dismiss Ross "would damage the reputation of the University in the eyes of the academic community" and that Ross had "already been censured by me for his indiscretions" (Curti and Cartenson, 1949, p. 146). The regents censured but did not dismiss Ross. It is reasonable to believe that support of academic freedom for social scientists went along with increasing academic freedom for physical and biological scientists. University subjects were shifting from classical education, with its pervasive religious component, to scientific education, with its secular component. To have dismissed Ross (or, earlier, Ely) would perhaps have been seen as threatening the more established sciences as well. The retention of Ross may have been a watershed in academic freedom at the University of Wisconsin, for the issue did not seem to come up again. The university kept and strengthened its liberal reputation ever after. The activities of social scientists—particularly those of John R. Commons with respect to regulation of what he regarded as rampant and irresponsible capitalism—are an enduring if attenuated legacy at the university to this day.

Thus, by the time John L. Gillin came on the scene, he was free to busy himself intensively with problems of crime and public welfare, under the rubric of social pathology. He became a national and international figure in social reform (particularly in criminology) within the democratic-capitalistic structure. His approach was, by comparison with current sociology, very normative; he had no doubt about what a good individual or a good society was, and he had no theory of pathology (what was later called *deviance*).

All the Wisconsin scholars mentioned so far were products of a particular period of American history. They came from very modest circumstances, from farms and villages, with a tremendous faith in education and in social reform based on systematically collected data. They were Protestants steeped in the belief in continual human and social progress. As social scientists, they accepted a moral obligation to improve society. With the exception of Gillin, they were hardly regular churchgoers, but the values of good works, personal responsibility, and hard work persisted in them. These academics were very popular among clergy in the Social Gospel movement.

By the 1920s, the field of social problems had become institutionalized in departments of sociology all over the country, usually in courses called Social Pathology or Social Problems. Many textbooks were published and adopted for these courses. The books were mainly descriptive in style, and they did not endeavor to conceptualize theories of social pathology or social problems. The causes of these problems were held to be self-evident: poverty, deficient education (both in morals and in skills), and an economic system that exploited labor. The exploiters were "bad" rather than "good" capitalists. They would become good capitalists through governmental regulation, just as citizens would become good citizens through education in the good society. Crime and greed would then diminish, and social engineering, carried out by means of the social sciences, would create a better society.

This view was embodied in a conservative Republican president, Herbert Hoover. He believed in the capitalist economy and in democracy (sovereignty of the people). An eminent engineer, who had faith in the power of assembled facts to improve economic planning and foster progress in all aspects of society, he shared the prevailing belief that rational people of good will, made more rational by the appropriate assemblage of facts bearing on problems, would implement policies leading to more production, more distribution, more profits, and more personal income. This was, in short, a technocratic and ostensibly apolitical view.

In 1929, Hoover appointed the still famous President's Research Committee on Social Trends (which submitted its report in 1933, after Hoover was no longer president). It is significant that the committee's director of research was William F. Ogburn, a sociologist at the University of Chicago who by this time had made his reputation as an empirical sociologist with a strong positivist bent. Ogburn studied social change, and his major independent variable was the geometric accumulation of technology, which was reshaping a rural society along industrial lines. The chairman of the committee was Wesley C. Mitchell, an economist of business-cycle fame. The committee's social science staff was stellar. The staff produced, in one enormous tome, chapters on social trends in the United States from the latter nineteenth century to the early 1930s, transportation, food production, industrial development, increased educational attainment of the people, crime, poverty, divorce, marriage, health levels—all indicators of material and moral progress. The concept of proper morals was implicit, a given; the rising divorce rate, for example, was socially pathological by definition. This report afforded wide publicity to Ogburn's famous concept of "cultural lag." Ogburn had theorized that technology caused uneven advances and changes in the social system, subparts of which did not adjust as they should have to automobiles, electricity, labor-saving devices, and so on. The report beautifully reflected the received values of the time, of which Hoover the engineer and Ogburn the sociologist were ideal representatives. This report (President's Research Committee on Social Trends, 1933) was published shortly before I became interested in sociology and social problems. It seemed to pervade our academic thinking about society and social problems, instilling and reinforcing concepts that I later had to rethink, as I shall describe.

Raising of the "Value-Free" Issue

By the 1940s, there began to emerge another generation of scholars, who were attempting to conceptualize a theory of social problems. Simultaneously, or very soon thereafter, sociologists began to debate the concept of a value-free social science, the kernel of which was formulated by Max Weber early in the century (in a German university and a German economic and political context).

The three leaders of the Wisconsin School, like the German academic social-political economists, did not question the theoretical basis of prevailing concepts of the good society. Max Weber was a contemporary of them all, and congenial to their liberal-democratic values, but he apparently had not yet influenced their habit of taking their values as givens. Weber's work on the "value-free" concept was not published until shortly after World War I. Among sociologists who were paying any attention at all to theoretical orientation as it affects theories of society and of social problems, Weber's work (Runciman and Matthews, 1978, pp. 69–98) began to stimulate debate on this problem, peculiar to social science in this country.

The question that Weber raised was whether, in the academic and scholarly context, the professor's value judgments ought or ought not to be acknowledged. Such judgments may be based on ethical standards, cultural ideals, or other kinds of world view. Weber wrote that the question cannot even be discussed in scientific terms, because it is itself entirely dependent on practical value judgments and is therefore unresolvable; but, given these qualifications, Weber espoused value-free social research. The opposite view, of course, was taken by Karl Marx, who asserted that value judgments were inherent in the analytical process. The important point here, in any case, is that my generation of social science students at the University of Wisconsin–Madison was not put upon by the professors to stretch its minds with such abstract epistemological questions.

After Weber, the Swedish social economist Gunnar Myrdal was one of the first to write about the problem of the relationship between social action and theory. He also pointed out that the early reformers in the social sciences thought of values as a given—as, in effect, an independent variable. Social policy had been their primary interest, and social theory was secondary. As Myrdal wrote (and as many have observed since), "We stand continuously before research tasks where a clash of interests and valuations is part of the problem" (Streeten, 1958, p. 9).

Almost as a casual comment on the problem of values and action, Walter Lippmann, as early as 1914 (even earlier, when we consider how long it takes a book to be published), and apparently without being noticed by the social scientists, struck at the heart of this problem in describing the research approach of the Chicago Vice Commission. Lippmann says that the commission, in its efforts to shape policies, did not seek a theory of social reform and society but rather sought out what would "pass for moral, practical, popular, or constitutional." He continues, "In this, the [Chicago] Vice Commission reflected our national habits. For those earnest men and women in Chicago did not set out to find a way of abolishing prostitution; they set out to find a way that would conform to four idols they worshiped. The only cure for prostitution might prove to be 'immoral,' 'impractical,' unconstitutional, and unpopular. I suspect it is. But the honest thing to do would have been to look for that cure without preconceived notions. Having found it, the Commission could then have said to the public: 'This is what will cure the social evil. It means these changes in industry, sex relations, law and public opinion. If you think it is worth the cost you can begin to deal with the problem. If you don't, then confess that you will not abolish prostitution and turn your compassion to softening its effects'" (Lippmann, 1914, p. 172). Social reformers today seem to continue to hold completely malleable concepts of human beings and social systems, as if all the desirable elements will remain constant while the undesirable ones disappear. There is always a trade-off, however, and the acceptance of a net result, somewhere between values and interests, continues to be controversial. The abortion, AIDS, and drug questions are all rife with incompatible objectives and methods.

Late in the 1930s, Richard C. Fuller, a lawyer and sociologist at the University of Michigan, began to open up the social scientific conceptualization of the idea of a social problem. To see a problem in this way, Fuller said, social scientists had to detach themselves from their own definition of it. They also had to regard values as objects that were as real as the social conditions toward which those values were directed: "The core of the social problem is a multi-sided clash of social interests. The job of the sociologist is to isolate and define these conflicting value judgments which are the *modus operandi* of the problem" (Fuller, 1938, p. 145). John L. Gillin, asked to write a rejoinder to this statement, seemed not to understand what Fuller meant. Gillin wrote that people should change their attitudes and come to agreements, in order to have a smoothly functioning society. Gillin was my mentor at the time, and I was not even aware of the controversy; I had completely absorbed the social science reformers' concepts of society and social problems, concepts dating from fifty years before.

When I left Wisconsin, in 1938, for the University of Michigan (where, in passing, I earned a B.A. in library science), I was exposed to theoretical thinking about social reform. I took a course from Fuller. By 1941, Fuller had elaborated his concept of the social problem with a colleague, Richard R. Myers: "A social problem is a condition which is an actual or imagined deviation from some social norm cherished by a considerable number of persons. But who is to say whether a condition is such a deviation? The sociologist may say so, but that does not make the condition a social problem from the standpoint of the layman" (Fuller and Myers, 1941, p. 25). To put it in shorthand, social problems are what people think they are. "In contrast to the physical problem at the first level, the ameliorative problem is truly 'social' in that sense that it is a man-made condition. By this we mean that value-judgments not only help to create the condition, but to prevent its solution" (Fuller and Myers, 1941, p. 29). This is what Lippmann had been trying to explain.

Thirty years later, Blumer (1971, p. 299) revisits the concept of the social problem and seems to take off from Fuller and Myers, but he adds that "current sociological theory and knowledge, in themselves, just do not enable detection or identification of social problems. Instead, sociologists discern problems only *after* they are recognized as social problems by and in society."

The early reformers already discussed here simply did not (and probably even could not) think in these terms. There are still sociologists on the left-liberal end of the political spectrum, not to mention Marxists, who refuse to conceptualize in these terms, and who deny the possibility of detaching themselves from problems for analytical purposes. Indeed, they even appear to feel it is pernicious to do so. They seem to argue that they are policymakers as legitimate as politicians or interest groups. In this connection, Glazer (1967, p. 67) takes to task the radical critics of society who speak as sociologists because "even the most scientific parts of sociology— its most abstruse methodology, its most abstract theory—can be and are regularly brought under attack by some sociologists as ideology, as serving some social and political end by obscuring the social reality of society." This was written in the 1960s—the heyday, it will be recalled, of the rhetoric of left-liberal, radical sociologists; perhaps Glazer's statement is not so true today. To quote Glazer again, this time on the sociology of health, "When we say the sociology of health, we mean the part that shows that doctors and nurses are moved by prestige and status rather than simply the needs of the patient" (p. 75), and "the illusions that sociology is most heir to are not the illusion of the established and the establishment, but the illusion that life is a fraud, that men never mean what they say, and that institutions are never devoted to their ostensible ends. Now, while all this is true to some extent, to maximize such views is to shape an ideology" (p. 76).

There are sociologists who believe that they should play a prophetic role in moving toward a concept of the good society (one in which poverty is eliminated and the distance between those who have little and those who have much is narrowed); that there should be pure participatory democracy, so that individuals have some say in decisions that affect them directly and indirectly; that people reach public decisions on the basis of facts; that decisions are rationally implemented; and so on. However desirable the good society may seem, it is essentially utopian; it can only be approximated. It assumes an extremely narrow range of value consensus, with very little deviation, and even this must be curbed (and the deviants perhaps liquidated). The degree to which this ideal is approximated could be a concern of social and psychological science, but the concept of an *approximate* level of attainment does not seem to interest sociologists, by and large; it is too pessimistic. Still, every attempt at approaching utopia must involve net results and trade-offs. Horowitz and Katz (1975), for example, write eloquently and wistfully about a concept of the good society, an ideal that our current political and economic systems seem far from attaining. They observe (p. 38) that the sociologist becomes enmeshed in fact gathering of the "social indicator" type and becomes a technician for the existing order: "He gets caught up in the theoryless applications to immediate problems, surrenders the value of confronting men with an image of what can be and simply accepts what others declare must be." Waitzkin (1968) writes that for the social scientist there is a tension between the optimistic assumption that scientific rationality can solve social problems and the realistic observation that he himself lacks power; therefore, he wants power. If sociologists get power, however, Waitzkin predicts that they will and must behave as all politicians do. They will compromise, or they will liquidate their opponents.

In my view, Bellah (1983, pp. 63-64), within his prophetic mission, comes close to a practical view of sociologists who wish to be active in social reform: "Practical social scientists do not claim the degree cf scientific precision to which technological social science aspires. Partly because they do not think it possible in the study of human affairs. This means that there is a considerable humility in their claims. They do not offer definitive findings but only judgments informed by inquiry, quite fallible and containing many links that cannot be conclusively demonstrated. In this practical social scientists do not claim to be strikingly different from or superior to those who are addressed, whether ordinary citizens or decision makers. Such scientists see themselves precisely within the process of practical reason, where prudence and judgment must operate because scientific demonstration is not possible." Kai Nielsen (1983, p. 128) elaborates Bellah's observations: "There is, of course, little point in talking about the 'should' unless we have an understanding of the 'can.' " In other words, according to Nielsen, sociology should be a science, taking the Enlightenment rather than social engineering as a model.

Perhaps the "value-free–value-laden" controversy has now been presented clearly enough for me to go on to some observations of and experiences with the social scientists who have wandered into applied social science. To one degree or another, they and I have experienced the slings and arrows of conducting social research that sometimes displeases various interest groups.

My own values, I believe, are evident in the foregoing paragraphs. I have to believe in the premise of an objective reality, which has its own order or disorder apart from the observer; otherwise, a social science at any level of abstraction is impossible. Social scientists have become more skillful at dissecting the components of social problems in social and ideological contexts, and they are able to predict, with some degree of plausibility, the results of various alternatives for achieving given ends by given means. Certainly, we are learning more about the nature of social systems in that we now recognize incompatible objectives and the need for rational trade-offs. My values will continue to be discernible in my behavior, which I shall describe as I interpret the development of my research career in the chapters that follow.

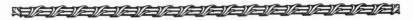

2

"Solving"
Social Problems with
Social Research:
Four Classic Examples

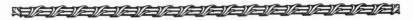

Social research results may be ignored, attacked, or welcomed, according to the nature of the issues and the perceptions of the interest groups who are implicated. A useful classification scheme, suggested by Sol Levine, is that some research has political implications, to the extent that the results are ignored or attacked; some research results may threaten the products of commercial interests; and some results are eagerly welcomed because they are wanted by many parties at the same time (telephone interview with Sol Levine, October 31, 1988). I might add another classification, which cuts across these three: sometimes research has implications for research design and methodology and sparks debate among methodologists so that those who dislike the results may attack the research on grounds of deficient methodology.

It behooves researchers to be fully conscious of the issues and interests their research will affect and to be formulating their responses at the same time that funding sources are being sought, projects selected, research designs formulated, results written up, audiences addressed, and findings disseminated. This perspicacity would seem to be the essence of applied research directed to social problems; research designed to contribute to social theory would be much less concerned with such external factors, because funding sources and peer evaluation of theory would be the dominant concerns.

The social scientists discussed in this chapter were selected because of their experiences with applied research. They were responsive to the social problems that concerned them as citizens. They wanted to draw on social science concepts, theory, and methodology to understand and solve social problems as social and political processes. At best, they were conceptualizing theories of implementation and problem solving. As will be seen, some of their research became very controversial. They rubbed the raw nerves of some interest groups and were attacked by research colleagues and interest groups alike. They also endured a great deal of simplistic publicity in the media because the controversies they aroused were newsworthy.

In some cases, controversy was limited to a narrow range of interest groups and methodologists, and the research was publicized only in trade and professional journals. In other cases, when there was consensus among many parties that problems needed solutions, controversy over research results focused sometimes on data that seemed to exaggerate the severity of a problem and sometimes on data that seemed to understate it.

I selected four cases from the early 1960s to the early 1980s because this period includes the tempestuous War on Poverty period of the Johnson administration and the era of the Vietnam War; later would come the problems of the uninsured and homeless and the rapidly escalating cost of health services. My own research starts fifteen or so years earlier and encompasses the early 1980s. I started in a research position at the University of Michigan School of Public Health in 1942, when the most controversial public policy issue concerned compulsory government-funded health insurance versus private (or, as it was called, voluntary) health insurance. The two polar concepts were fraught with ideological overtones. (The other public problem at that time, of course, was winning the war with Japan and Germany, which had the full backing of Congress and the American people. World War II showed what a country could do when it was united behind a policy.) Moving into health services research, as I did, marked one as a proponent of compulsory health insurance; otherwise, one would not be interested in research into health insurance plans or in related activities. The most controversial research and researchers between the 1960s and the 1980s, however, were not involved at all with health-related issues. The examples presented here were selected because of the intense conflicts among researchers and between researchers and interest groups. Nevertheless, these cases do serve as a context for health services research because they touch on value-laden issues of race (in terms of civil rights and racial equality). Another problem of this period, reflected in one of the cases discussed here, was the role of the U.S. government in foreign countries' internal political affairs. It seemed to be mainline social scientists, especially sociologists, who were engaged in research on the burning issues of that time. By *mainline* I mean those who more or less took for granted the liberal-democratic interest-group political process—the basic concepts of Western liberal democracies. They were liberals (in the American sense of the word), as are the great majority of sociologists, but they leaned toward the left in their tendency to believe in an active role for government in human affairs.

The Moynihan Report

The published results of the first of the four research projects discussed in this chapter became known as the Moynihan Report. It was an in-house position paper from the Department of Labor's Office of Policy and Research and was prepared by the assistant secretary of labor, Daniel Patrick Moynihan (now the Democratic senator from New York). The paper was released internally in March 1965 (Rainwater and Yancy, 1967). It reported on the condition of black families in America, particularly in the inner cities. On June 4, 1965, President Johnson gave the commencement address at Harvard University, in which he focused on the economic condition of blacks. The president's speech uncovered the existence of this report on an explosive political issue, a report produced by a very visible government agency. Had the report been produced independently (by a scholar in a university, for example), it probably would not have started the prairie fire that it did. Unfortunately, the report came into the public domain only after the press had publicized its contents. Politicians, policymakers, and the interested public had no other source of information about it than simplified accounts in daily newspapers and news broadcasts. This report, reposing in the bowels of a massive bureaucracy, caused a storm of public controversy: "From the anonymous layers of the federal government, in the inner councils of some civil rights groups, in unpublished memoranda and private denunciations, in the professional conversations of some social scientists, and finally, in public meetings and in the press the report (but not the President's speech) increasingly came under attack during the later summer and fall of the year [1965]" (Rainwater and Yancy, 1967, p. 4). The Johnson administration had established the framework for political civil rights, and now some attention was being paid to economic rights. Black families in inner cities, of course, were a very visible target of efforts to help. Given Moynihan's relatively high position in the government, the report had serious policy implications for the administration.

The report stressed family interests, especially those of the traditional nuclear family (recall that this was twenty-six years ago). Moynihan felt that emphasis should be on employment, income maintenance, and education and (perhaps because of his Catholic background) that the policy focus should be on the stability of the family—that is, support of the nuclear family. Other social scientists felt that the report should have stressed the adaptation and coping mechanisms—the strengths—of inner-city families. The report's explicit value bias was toward the conventional middle-class family model. Further, the report implicated all black families. Women's groups attacked the report because it assumed that men should be heads of families, and so on and on. Moynihan produced reams of census data showing the comparatively high proportion of households headed by single mothers, high birthrates among unmarried mothers, and high rates of juvenile delinquency. Some critics felt that the victims were being blamed, instead of society.

I do not believe that Moynihan was really as naïve as he was made to seem. He was aware of conflicting and incompatible values. Understandably enough, he took modern industrial society and the American political process as givens—as practical if not ideological matters. The concept of transforming society to fit the inner-city culture (rather than changing the inner-city culture so that it could function better in society) was hardly an option.

The welfare establishment was also in a very difficult position because it should have known better than anyone else how inadequate the national welfare programs were. At the same time, this establishment was responsible for carrying out and defending those programs against political attacks from all sides. The report was too "alarming" for the welfare establishment, and it was too "optimistic" for civil rights groups (Rainwater and Yancy, 1967, pp. 175-176).

The central issue, according to Rainwater and Yancy (1967), is that the report was basically not a research report or even a technical document; it was a legitimate polemic within the established political process of policymaking. It used carefully derived findings to make a political point, through research prepared for and funded by an administration whose policy was to ameliorate poverty, especially among blacks in the inner cities, and Moynihan maintained high technical standards.

Later, Moynihan wrote a book quite critical of social scientists' behavior during the heyday of President Johnson's poverty program. In his preface, he observes: "We constantly underestimate difficulties, overpromise results, and avoid any evidence of incompatibility and conflict, thus repeatedly creating the conditions of failure out of a desperate desire for success" (Moynihan, 1969, p. xii). Moynihan (and he is not alone) believes that social scientists know too little about social processes to be able to manipulate relationships within social systems for desired ends. He concludes (p. 193) that "the role of social science lies not in the formulation of social policy [by people as social scientists] but in the measurement of its results." This role may seem too modest for social scientists, whose evaluation skills are improving. Nevertheless, even the results of evaluations become controversial.

The Coleman Reports

A report initiated by the U.S. Office of Education and known as one of the Coleman Reports (Coleman and others, 1966) dealt with the very controversial issue of school desegregation. It was directed by a well-regarded academic sociologist, James S. Coleman, at that time in the Department of Sociology at Johns Hopkins University. According to Gerald Grant (1973), this report had rather obscure origins in the Civil Rights Act of 1964, which was conceived in the Kennedy administration, only to languish in Congress before finally being enacted in the traumatic days after President Kennedy's assassination (in part as a testament to him). At the time, the section of the bill authorizing what eventually became the first Coleman Report received no notice. Public attention focused mainly on the voting-rights and public-accommodations titles of the bill. Section 402 stressed blacks' lack of access to adequate education.

The U.S. Office of Education did not want an inventory of school buildings, equipment, and books, the usual evaluation variables, but rather a classroom-based study of verbal and mathematical skills. This was an unprecedented step, which involved the Office of Education for the first time in the politically sensitive sponsorship of classroom testing. Even a decade earlier, such a survey would not have been considered; the Office of Education had not dared ask "how well anyone was doing with what they had" (Grant, 1973, p. 19).

The Office of Education was impressed by Coleman's previous work and by his ability to handle a large social survey. Survey research methodology was also being greatly improved by the use of computers. Coleman was engaged as an outside contractor and consultant, rather than as an Office of Education employee. This was obviously a wise tactical move, to distance the Office of Education from the research, since the bureaucracy feared political backlash should the findings turn out to be controversial.

The survey was massive, by any standard. Around 600,000 children completed tests of verbal and mathematical ability and filled out questionnaires on details of their environment and economic status. Teachers, 60,000 of them, were also queried about school facilities and environments. Coleman expected the opposite of what he found. He expected variation in school resources to have the greatest impact on the relative performance of black and white children. Instead, he found that variation in family resources had a greater impact on achievement (Barber, 1987, p. 38).

Later studies (published in the 1970s) showed that, to various degrees, the busing of black children to predominantly white schools was a factor in whites' flight to the suburbs. This research (a series of progress reports) also came to be called the Coleman Report. It was funded by the Urban Institute. The report was vigorously dissected from a methodological standpoint by Pettigrew and

Green (1976). Probably no other piece of sociological research on any problem has been so intensively critiqued by other sociologists. These critics were strong advocates of busing as a method of integrating public schools. Coleman's report cast doubt on the method's efficacy, since he interpreted his findings as showing that busing caused "white flight." Pettigrew and Green rather cogently argued that busing itself was only one of the factors (and a minor one, at that) in the massive migration of white middle-class families from the cities to the suburbs, leaving large sections of the inner cities to a black underclass. According to Pettigrew and Green, the busing study should have been carried out in a larger context, both longitudinally and cross-sectionally, because the white move to the suburbs was systemic. Official social policy was creating incentives: tax deductions for home mortgages and the construction of highways for quick and easy access to the suburbs (in fact, these highways cut through and virtually destroyed the lower- and middle-class urban neighborhoods that existed at that time).

Coleman participated in several formal critiques of his busing study, with apparent patience. According to Pettigrew and Green (1976, p. 50), he conducted himself in a "businesslike" way. A more serious criticism than the one involving his methodology concerned Coleman's straying from his data, by his own admission, in testimony given in Boston about the city's controversial busing mandate and in comments made to the press.

Controversy over this study was not laid to rest by the various critiques. Alfred McClung Lee, then president of the American Sociological Association (ASA), was very agitated by the report. He also felt that Coleman, as an academician, was engaging in behavior that constituted a serious breach of research integrity and of the use of social research findings in the name of sociology. Lee asked the ASA Council and the association's Committee on Professional Ethics "to give serious consideration to the unsubstantiated statements being made by James S. Coleman . . . before legislative, judicial, and other public forums." Lee said that Coleman's statements "presented findings against the use of busing for educational opportunity equalization," and that Coleman was using his findings in the name of sociology. In making his request, Lee referred to an ASA document that stated, "Sociology must not be an instrument of any person or group who seeks to . . . misuse knowledge" (Lee, 1986, p. 191). The ASA Council rejected Lee's request on the basis of Coleman's right to freedom of expression and conscience. Lee's answer was that freedom of expression and conscience was not the issue. Recalling the events a decade later, Lee wrote, "At the same time, I would not free Coleman from critical review by his fellow sociologists. I insist that his pouring of what amounted to flammable propaganda on the conflict situations in South Boston and in other American cities requires some judicious consideration by responsible agencies of our professional associations." Moreover, "freedom of expression does not mean freedom from criticism. Critical consideration of such matters is the least we can and should expect from sociologists in control of our professional association. We did not receive it" (Lee, 1986, pp. 191–192). Lee went farther and attempted to have Coleman censured at the annual ASA meeting in August 1976. To have one's methodology critiqued by colleagues is, of course, a normal process; to be censured for one's methodology is not. This attempt at censure was unprecedented in the ASA (and perhaps in any other professional scientific association) because it was founded on a critique of methodology and was an attack on Coleman's public interpretations of the study's results. Twelve years later, Coleman received the American Sociology Association's Willard Waller Award in Education. Recalling the earlier period of "intellectual isolation" and attacks, he said, "The passions generated at that session are hard to reconstruct now, but I still have the posters that were plastered at the entrance of the [hotel] ballroom and behind the podium covered with Nazi swastikas, epithets, and my name." Coleman went on to observe that the prevailing styles of research at that time had inhibited younger scholars from engaging in studies whose results might have been unpopular (Coleman, 1989, p. 4).

Let us return now to the critique by Pettigrew and Green, who make a master understatement: "This article has not been easy to write" (Pettigrew and Green, 1976, p. 5). (I too find this description of events, charges, and countercharges difficult to put in perspective.) They go on to say, "The information necessary to evaluate Coleman's much publicized research has been consistently difficult to obtain. Throughout the furor created by Coleman's statements, there has been confusion about where his limited research ends and his sweeping opposition to court-ordered desegregation begins. When critics questioned his views, they repeatedly suffered *ad hominem* abuse. Some critics have hurled such abuse at Coleman. We regret all such *ad hominem* remarks deeply" (Pettigrew and Green, 1976, p. 5). I assume that the display of swastikas and epithets at the 1976 ASA meeting was not the work of Pettigrew or Green but rather of extremists outside the control of methodological critics like them. Leggett (1989) raises a general question in research and public policy: Where do research-based generalizations applicable to the empirical universe end, and where do summary and political statements with a high degree of generality begin? Coleman himself has reported being surprised that government groups and implicated agencies seemed to take little direct interest in any of his three studies; most of the results of the desegregation studies were used by the courts. The mass media did make much of the reports, but Coleman found "the mass media extraordinarily unsuited to the complexities of social research results" (cited in Barber, 1987, pp. 38, 39). Coleman concludes that what is most valuable in policy research is to show administrators (and anyone else involved in policy) how they need to change their conceptions of how the system works: "The role of social research is not to tell these people what policy to carry out. It should provide only one input to the process, to aid an understanding of how the system works, which might lead them to carry out policies they would not have tried before. I think we should promise much less direct effect . . . in policy making" (cited in Barber, 1987, p. 41). Coleman discovered that ideology and methodology were intertwined, but the methodological questions finally got resolved (except in the minds of Coleman's harshest critics—some of the most committed of whom, Coleman says, flatly refused to accept the possibility of negative results from a study of school desegregation).

In this connection, Daniel P. Moynihan makes an apt observation (certainly based on his own experiences): Coleman had taken on three establishments at once—the educational establishment, the reform establishment, and the research establishment. Each had its own predilections and its own style of operating, to which groundbreaking research constituted a latent threat (Moynihan, 1968). For Coleman, "social science . . . should not be the determining element in policy, but only one of a variety of inputs into policy decisions, and it should be an input that aids the pluralism or democracy of the policy process" (cited in Barber, 1987, p. 43). This view harks back to an old political aphorism: that experts should be on tap but not on top.

I have known James Coleman for many years, and I asked him if he had expected the uproar that his research results on busing evoked. His answer was no. Was he not, then, somewhat naïve? He said yes (interview with Coleman, November 6, 1988). Coleman's admitted naïveté is not peculiar to him, by any means, but his candor is unusual and commendable; it is unlikely that he has been so naïve since. His experience stands as an object lesson to social policy researchers: be sure of your methodology, and experiment with methodology on relatively noncontroversial problems. Of course, social scientists of all sorts make public policy statements, but usually not in the heat of ideological controversies surrounding race and equity. Economists, for example, make guarded or unguarded pronouncements all the time. In all good faith, I ask this question: If Coleman's research, using somewhat faulty methodology, had produced results favorable to the idea of busing as a method of integrating the public schools, would the proponents of busing have attacked Coleman's methodology?

Coleman made the tactical mistake of releasing his findings before his research was completed and in the public domain. He seemed to be improvising as he went along and releasing data in the process. This was a mistake because the findings, by their very nature, would have been controversial in any case.

Wilson and the Black American Underclass

In 1978, William J. Wilson, professor of sociology at the University of Chicago, published *The Declining Significance of Race: Blacks and Changing American Institutions*. In this book (widely publicized because it questioned the conventional wisdom), Wilson argued, using a mass of supporting data, that a black middle class had emerged, and that an isolated black underclass had thereby been created in the inner cities. Wilson held that there can be no black political movement per se because blacks, like any other interest group, are becoming differentiated within the class and occupational structures. One favorable review of the book called it a significant piece of research in political sociology and observed that it undermines the promise of racial solidarity: it inhibits the development of racial movements based on an overwhelming consensus regarding specific goals and their means of attainment and, what is probably most serious, it casts doubt on the ability and even the right of black leaders to speak for blacks as a group. The review went on to say that Wilson's book will induce blacks to view themselves as members of different socioeconomic classes who have noncomplementary (if not conflicting) interests, rather than as members of an oppressed minority who have a shared past and a common culture (Record, 1980).

In the same month (January 1980) that this favorable review was published, Thomas F. Pettigrew, one of the most severe critics of the Coleman Report on busing, wrote an unfavorable review. He wrote that Wilson's book, "weak theoretically," was "a useful though premature start." He criticized the title as political: "I believe . . . the chief conclusion of this volume—the declining significance of race—to be premature at best, dangerously wrong at worst. The unqualified title draws attention to the book. . . . In the politically charged arena of race relations, [Wilson's] misleading title has already been exploited by conservative spokesmen" (Pettigrew, 1980, p. 21).

The book was reviewed in virtually every major social science journal: *Annals of American Political and Social Science, American Political Science Review, Dissent, Social Forces,* and *Sociological Review.* There may have been other reviews as well. One might have expected the review in *Dissent* to be critical, but the reviewer called the book a "sophisticated" treatment of the black inner-city ghetto and merely suggested that Wilson had paid too little attention to continuing institutional racism in the United States, which probably influenced employment opportunities—a reasonable enough criticism, which had also been made by other reviewers (Kennedy, 1979). A review by Martin (1980) in the *American Political Science Review* was also very favorable.

Nine years later, Wilson published another book (Wilson, 1987b), elaborating his thesis that inner-city blacks should be regarded as a low-income class, along with white low-income groups, because their problems were low-income problems, rather than race-related problems. Inner-city blacks, Wilson wrote, have basically the same problems as other low-income groups, problems caused by the movement in America and other postindustrial countries away from heavy industry and toward light and service industries. This new book, *The Truly Disadvantaged: The Inner City, the Underclass, and Public Policy*, was given an essentially favorable review in *Contemporary Sociology*— although, again, the reviewer said that Wilson had not paid enough attention to institutional racism (Duster, 1988). In my estimation, Duster is right when he says, "This book is a major statement on public policy and race relations in the United States, and it will be widely influential in shaping the discourse about that policy" (p. 287). Duster also recognizes the vortex of which Wilson has become the center: "Broadly conceived, there are three major competing theories or schools of thought on race in America. Wilson turns his analytic guns on two of the three. First, he takes on the liberals, whom he sees as floundering around with an antiquated and 'simple' theory of race discrimination, unable to handle the searing white-hot truth of inner-city urban blight" (p. 287). (He also sees some responses to the Moynihan Report as embodying a mindless, misguided, mean-spirited attack on researchers who have dared to touch this topic and tell the truth as they see it.) According to Duster, Wilson then "takes on the conservatives, criticizing them for not understanding that the affliction of the inner city cannot be explained by looking only internally at the qualities of the residents of those areas. Contrary to the conservative litany, he presents a compelling argument and strong supporting data to demonstrate that joblessness, not welfare dependency, is at the heart of black family disintegration" (p. 287).

The 1987 book seems to have brought Wilson to the attention of both the conservative and the liberal establishment news media, not to mention the other professional journals. The *New Yorker* reviewed it, as did the *New York Review of Books*, the *National Review*, the *New Republic*, the *New York Times*, *Commentary*, and *Dissent*, among others.

The review in *Dissent* (Bensman, 1988) was even more favorable than Wilson's previous review in that magazine. The reviewer observed that Wilson was taking on everybody: blacks, liberals, and neoconservatives. Another favorable review, in the *New Republic* (Jencks, 1988), was also an elaborate and thoughtful essay on the underclass in the United States. Jencks called Wilson an "academic radical," a "cultural conservative," and a "political pragmatist." Presumably, Jencks called Wilson an academic radical for being bold enough to tackle, in a scholarly fashion, a thorny and politically controversial problem; a cultural conservative for pointing out the influence of culture on human behavior; and a political pragmatist for seeing social improvements as possible only within the traditional American political process. Jencks also wrote, "Wilson's greatest contribution may be his discussion of how liberals' reluctance to blame blacks for anything that is happening in the communities has clouded both black thinking and white thinking about how we can improve these communities" (p. 32). In any case, the title of this book—*The Truly Disadvantaged*—was not criticized as pandering to conservatives, as was the title *The Declining Significance of Race;* the second title was seen as starkly descriptive.

The reviewer for the *National Review* (Klinghoffer, 1988) took the hard conservative line: that Wilson was "soft on black culture." The reviewer wrote that Wilson wanted desperately to distance himself from the "culture of poverty" thesis—the idea that the easy availability of generous transfer payments has bred a culture of dependency among underclass blacks. "The old-style Great Society liberals," according to the reviewer, "were happy to throw money at the black underclass, hoping it would buy a new suit and join the middle class" (p. 48).

Commentary's reviewer (Mead, 1988) seems to reflect a similar ideology, but in less lively language. Mead writes that the book is a good description of the stark conditions of the black underclass, but the "collective measures" that Wilson recommends, "although they might help working people, will not avail those who fail to work. Even as hardheaded as Wilson is, he finally acquiesces in the orthodoxy among liberal analysts, which is to assign all the responsibility for social problems to society itself, none to the poor. From such reasonings, government derives a mandate only to manipulate surrounding conditions, but not to govern the poor themselves so as to enforce civility" (p. 48).

Finally, an anonymous reviewer in the *New Yorker* wrote cryptically, in a very short review, that "Wilson and his collaborators . . . have worked a miracle of common sense and delineated a policy for the next era of American reform" (Review of *The Truly Disadvantaged*, 1988, p. 124).

In November 1988, I had a long interview with Wilson, to get some idea of his thinking and experience, beyond his publications and reactions to them (see also O'Sullivan, 1989). Major criticisms of Wilson came from black sociologists, who accused him of "copping out" by not being an advocate for blacks. Wilson, however, feels that it is better sociological analysis (and more realistic public policy) to look at class, rather than race, given the current status of the poverty class in the United States, regardless of its racial or ethnic segments. He says that the Urban League, for example, is too caught up in its own organization; it has become too black-oriented, not sufficiently class-oriented to be effective. Wilson believes that he is riding the wave of America's conscience. He is in overwhelming demand as a consultant and speaker; the *New York Times* calls him frequently. He is a personage and a sociologist of his time, and it seems that he is consciously taking advantage of the reemerging political interest in the American underclass, whatever motivates this interest. (For example, the political drive to insure the uninsured exists for other reasons besides altruism; it is being led by service providers who must serve the poor but suffer increasing financial constriction.)

Wilson is a stellar example of what happens on those rare occasions when there is the possibility of upward mobility against adversity (given the right family setting and personal characteristics). His father was a miner who died at thirty-nine, when Wilson was twelve years old. Wilson and all his siblings went to college; he said his mother was the major influence on this accomplishment.

"Some scholars," Wilson says, "in an effort to avoid the appearance of 'blaming the victim' or to protect their work from charges of racism, simply ignore patterns of behavior that might be construed as stigmatizing to particular racial minorities." He observes that this practice is relatively recent. During the mid 1970s, such social scientists as Kenneth Clark, Daniel Patrick Moynihan, and Lee Rainwater were forthright in examining the cumulative effects of racial isolation and class subordination on inner-city blacks; Clark called the phenomenon "self-perpetuating pathology" (Wilson, 1987a, p. 4). Wilson cites the experience of Moynihan, who was attacked by blacks and liberals for his "unflattering" description of the black family in the urban ghetto, and says that Moynihan's experience dissuaded many other social scientists from choosing that type of research problem. Wilson believes that insecure nontenured and even tenured social science researchers do not want to get embroiled in controversy.

Wilson appears to be a calm, nonthreatening person; he dresses inconspicuously, according to old-style Great Society liberal tradition. I asked Wilson how he would classify himself, both politically and as a sociologist. He regards himself as a mainline "left-liberal" establishment sociologist, and this description probably fits most other sociologists in the United States, who tend to believe that government should be the major agency (apart from the private sector) to solve the problems of the American underclass, if they can be solved at all.

Camelot

The 1964 social research project called Camelot never did become a project, for it collided with the politics of the United States' role in the internal affairs of Latin American countries. Camelot also became enmeshed in the question of academic social scientists' role in helping the U.S. government with its foreign policy problems. During World War II, such questions never arose, because the evil specter of Hitler and the Nazis was so overwhelming and beyond debate that social scientists, not to mention physical scientists, threw themselves into the massive effort to destroy Nazism. Social scientists studied troop morale, esprit de corps, and methods of selecting the right person for the right function and waging psychological warfare. A social science classic by Samuel Stouffer called *The American Soldier* came out of this research that contributed to both social psychology and the war effort. By 1964, not even twenty years after the end of World War II, this country and the rest of the world were in new alignments, fighting political brushfires. The United States was inhibiting the emergence of insurgent forces in Latin America trying to overthrow dictatorships (according to many academic social scientists, particularly sociologists and anthropologists). The U.S. policy of supporting the status quo was largely due to the fear of policymakers in both parties that imperialistic communism was trying to get footholds in the Western hemisphere.

In this explosive context, the U.S. Army's Special Operations Research Office (SORO) conceived the idea of making the most massive research grant ever proposed to social scientists up to that time, to help the military understand the social and political systems in Latin America, so that it could wage strategic war (or peace, as the case might be). The researchers were to conduct a social systems analysis of the origin and nature of insurgency; the feasibility study alone would cost $6 million.

A major source of information on these events is the extensive hearings initiated by the Committee on Foreign Affairs of the House of Representatives, held in 1965 (U.S. Congress, 1966). The hearings report:

> During recent years, Communist support of "wars of national liberation," and U.S. commitments to aid the developing nations of the free world to meet this threat, propelled our military establishment into an expanding involvement in research related to foreign areas and foreign populations. Noting the extent of this involvement, the Director of Defense Research and Engineering of the Department of Defense on April 24, 1964, requested the Defense Science Board to conduct a study of Defense research and development programs "relating to ethnic and other motivational factors involved in the causation and conduct of small wars***" [asterisks in the original]. The report produced by that study disclosed various deficiencies in the behavioral sciences research program of the Department of Defense. Among others, the report cited the need to improve "the knowledge and understanding in depth of the internal cultural, economic and political conditions that generate conflicts between

national groups," urged increased emphasis on the collections of initial primary data in overseas locations, and criticized The Military Establishment for "failure to organize appropriate multidisciplinary programs and to use the technologies of such related fields as operations research" [p. 3R].

To continue and paraphrase, since the Department of the Army was responsible for administering the military assistance program, as well as for research, planning, and organization for counterinsurgency and limited wars, the department initiated action on what became known as Project Camelot. The army then began to work through a contractor, SORO, at American University. The army sought to have a project formulated that would integrate many disparate research problems, to pursue a single operational objective and thus formulate a generalized model of a developing society, one evolving from basically agricultural to industrial society and, in this case, to be based on a Western democratic model. To quote again at length, in order to preserve the exact wording:

> The purpose of this project was to produce a better understanding of how the processes of change operate in the developing countries. On the one hand, Project Camelot was intended to assist in identifying the forerunners of social breakdown and the resultant opportunity for Communist penetration and possible takeover; on the other hand, it was also expected to produce basic information which would furnish some guidelines with respect to actions that might be taken by or with the indigenous governments to foster constructive change within a framework of relative order and stability [p. 3R].

To continue paraphrasing, the first phase of Project Camelot (which was to have been completed in the summer of 1964) was concentrated on developing the research design and recommendations for where the field work should be done. The preliminary proposals were to be submitted for review by the army's research staff, the Department of Defense, and other government agencies, including the Department of State. With their recommendations and approval, the actual research work was to start either late in 1965 or in 1966. When its existence became known, however, Project Camelot never went beyond the first phase.

While the preparatory work was in progress, a SORO representative, who was going to Chile on personal business, attempted in passing to gauge interest and available resources in that country: Would researchers in Chile like to be included in plans for the program and the research design? This SORO representative had absolutely no power to negotiate or make commitments. He was a naturalized American, formerly a Chilean citizen. He knew Chile and its research resources, but he made a mistake by acting informally; there might be leaks. Indeed, a leak did come from another source: SORO had sent a preliminary draft of the research proposal and design to social scientists all over the world. One was a Norwegian sociologist, Johan Galtung of Oslo, who was on the staff of Oslo's International Peace Research Institute and was living in Chile, working as a UNESCO professor (Horowitz, 1967, p. 283). A Chilean colleague (or colleagues) of Galtung's released information on the project to Chilean newspapers, including *El Siglo,* a reportedly Communist organ. Criticism of Project Camelot was hardly limited to the Communists. As the hearings report, "A distorted version of . . . [the SORO representative's] activities and of the project appeared in a local newspaper, reported to be pro-Communist, and led to considerable adverse publicity in Chile, elsewhere abroad, and in the United States. The American Ambassador to Chile, having no previous knowledge of Project Camelot, protested to Washington and the resulting furor prompted the Army to cancel the project on August 2, 1965" (U.S. Congress, 1966, p. 4R). President Lyndon Johnson also ordered that no research implicating the foreign policy of the United States be started without the approval of the Department of State. The members of the House Committee on Foreign Affairs were by no means naïve about the sponsorship of research in foreign countries, particularly when it was tied to military intelligence. According to the hearings, "as the recent experience with Project Camelot has demonstrated, some U.S. research efforts can provoke extremely unfavorable reactions abroad not only from the Communists and their sympathizers but *also from academic and political groups that are generally friendly to the United States* [my emphasis]. There exists in every country a sensitivity to foreigners probing into delicate social and political matters. Also, the level of sensitivity varies according to who does the research and its subject matter" (p. 5R).

In this connection, Donald M. Fraser, a member of the House Committee on Foreign Affairs, was particularly sensitive. When Dr. Theodore Vallance, director of SORO at American University, indicated by his testimony that he was not fully aware of the extreme sensitivity among foreign countries toward Project Camelot, Fraser observed, "I suppose what this [foreign sensitivity] suggests is a need for an increased degree of caution and sensitivity to the rights—the fact that these are independent sovereign nations, that we have to be considerate of that fact."

Vallance replied, "Or at least heightened sensitivity to the possibility of encountering skeptical attitudes within the country that might misunderstand or, if they chose to, distort."

Fraser was not quite satisfied with Vallance's answer:

Yes, I must say this is not a problem that falls in your lap because you are carrying out an assignment at the request of our Government, but there is throughout your whole presentation a kind of an implicit attitude or relationship that this country bears to the rest of the world which, if I were not an American, I would find highly offensive, but it suggests somehow we are the ones to find out the dynamisms that are at work in these countries in their societies for the benefit of our Military Establishment. If I were a Latin American, I wouldn't find this a particularly happy arrangement. Our military assistance programs are primarily in the hardware field, although we also finance some of these civic action programs. Should this [Project Camelot] be the entering wedge to the study of the processes of development, the cultural changes and breakdowns and so on? Should this be the entering wedge for this kind of basic research? This suggests to me there is

something wrong. Not on your part because you are
doing a job, but in terms of the assignment or
allocation of responsibilities within our Government
[U.S. Congress, 1965, p. 17].

The members of the House Committee on Foreign Affairs, in
querying witnesses on Project Camelot, appeared very aware of the
international and internal political implications of the kind of research intended for the would-be project. Project Camelot was not
simply going to compile a sort of tourist handbook for servicemen;
it was going to reveal more about a particular society than its
members knew themselves, and this knowledge was going to be in
the hands of a foreign power. In principle, the members of Congress
were in favor of social and behavioral research, but Fraser, for one,
was dismayed that the military was behind Project Camelot; too
often, the United States was accused of supporting the status quo.
The army's chief of research and development defended the army's
position, saying that it had to make long-range predictions about
conditions of unrest in countries where the military could be ordered to move (U.S. Congress, 1965, p. 39).
    Secretary of State Dean Rusk also testified in answer to
Fraser:

RUSK: I think, sir, some of the language that is used
in devising these research projects is unfortunate from
the point of view of the foreign listener.

FRASER: If we are going to have change [in coun-
tries], the question is how we can influence that
change in directions that will be ultimately beneficial
to those people.

RUSK: I think that what we are looking for, sir, is
stability coupled with progress under democratic institutions. The Alliance for Progress is a revolutionary
movement. The effort is to be sure that change occurs
within democratic institutions. I don't believe our colleagues in Defense would interpret that in another
way [p. 118].

Another major source of information is Horowitz (1967), whose book on the Project Camelot debacle included contributions from members of Congress, government officials, and SORO researchers. Horowitz's overview is certainly plausible (pp. 6–8):

1. The men and women who worked for Project Camelot felt the need for wide-ranging social science research, instead of the usual small-scale studies. They wanted a social science of "contemporary relevance." Most of the participants viewed Project Camelot as a legitimate opportunity to engage in unrestricted fundamental research, with comparatively generous funds. "Under such optimal conditions, these scholars tended not to look a gift horse in the mouth." As one participant said, "There was no desire to inquire too deeply as to the military source of the funds or the ultimate purpose of the project."

2. A number of participants felt that there was actually more freedom "under selective sponsored conditions to do fundamental research in a nonacademic environment than at a university or college." The Rand Corporation was mentioned and "was almost viewed as a society of Platonists permitted to search for truth on the part of the powerful. A Neoplatonist definition of the situation by the men on Camelot was itself a constant in all of the interviews that were conducted."

3. Many of the Camelot researchers were uncomfortable with military sponsorship, particularly given the contemporary American foreign policy of intervention. Their reaction, however, was that the army merely had to be educated: "The discipline and order embodied in an army could be channeled into the process of economic and social development in the United States as well as in many parts of the Third World."

4. Among the Camelot social scientists there was "a profound conviction of the perfectibility of mankind." This was "the Enlightenment syndrome."

5. The Camelot personnel were upset by social scientists who were not willing to try anything new. They considered themselves to be in the forefront of applied social science and saw little difference between scholarship engaged in the war against poverty and scholarship engaged in a war against violence.

6. None of the Project Camelot personnel viewed their role as spying, either for the United States or for anyone else, nor did any believe that the army would take their recommendations seriously. There was a "keener appreciation on the part of the directing members of Camelot neither to 'sell out' or 'cop out.' "

Summarizing, Horowitz wrote (p. 11):

> As is often the case, the explosion of a big event begins in unpredictable circumstances and in unlikely surroundings. The actual crisis over Camelot came to a boiling point as a result of a congruence of several events. . . . The "showdown" took place in Chile. . . . From there on, the Camelot story moved to Washington: demands for a hearing, outcries from congressional figures, pained expressions of grief by State Department officials, revanchist sentiments of anger by the Defense Department officials, confusion by military intellectuals, and finally, the official announcement and resolution of the problem by Presidential epistle.

As Horowitz points out, one of the things that characterized Project Camelot was the amount of antagonism it inspired on grounds other than the quality of its research design. The project was attacked more in terms of strategic issues and timing, and "the mystique of social science seemed to have been taken for granted by friends and foes . . . alike" (p. 17). I understand Horowitz to mean that Camelot's critics seemed to overestimate the capacity of social and behavioral science to carry out, conceptually and methodologically, the ambitious objectives of such a project. My impression from the hearings is that Congress also took for granted the project's ability to deliver what seems to have been promised. In this regard, Horowitz himself is certainly very critical and modest about our current scientific ability to carry out studies of complex social forces. In his view, Project Camelot was intellectually and ideologically unsound. Nevertheless, Camelot was not canceled because of its deficient design; political expediency was the reason. A concluding comment from Horowitz (p. 40) puts the project in an even larger human perspective: "The story of Camelot was not a confrontation of good versus evil. Not that all men behaved with equal fidelity or with equal civility—that obviously was not the case. Some men were weaker than others; some more callous and some more stupid. But all this is extrinsic to the problem of Camelot. The heart of the question must always be, what are and are not the legitimate functions of a scientist?"

I shall conclude the story of Project Camelot here by citing an observer of (and, in a sense, a participant in) the problem of the social scientist and the military, Seymour J. Deitchman. Deitchman was an aeronautical engineer for defense problems and was interested in military affairs and strategy, and in the problems the U.S. military faces all over the world. He had been on the staff of the Institute for Defense Analysis since 1960. In October 1963, Deitchman was asked to join the Office of the Director of Defense Research and Engineering as special assistant to the secretary of the army. Deitchman told the secretary that the army had many important problems that required social science research, although the military and diplomats alike seemed to believe that conversations with a few villagers were enough to learn about a culture. Deitchman's book, published after the Project Camelot debacle, is a study of social research and bureaucratic cultures during the Camelot and Vietnam eras (Deitchman, 1976). His observation is that the question of social research sponsored by the military was initially understood as fundamentally an ethical issue: Were social scientists, by working on problems to help government achieve its objectives, violating their professional ethics? There seemed to be a view among social scientists that research aimed at avoiding violent political rebellion was reactionary, and that revolution should also be studied and supported as a necessary method of social change. Social scientists were much disturbed by the Vietnam War (Deitchman, 1976, pp. 255-256). Deitchman also observes that in the moral discourse in opposition to the Vietnam War, the buzzword was *dissent*: "If you were in dissent, you were 'concerned'; if you felt 'concern' you had to take an activist role, and become involved—against." In apparent criticism, Deitchman continues: "'Constancy'—a fundamental property of what earlier generations called 'character'—did not receive attention, or was rejected. If you felt the government was wrong, you should not try to help it change; you must oppose it. If a commitment had been made to help it, and government didn't instantly follow your advice, the commitment should instantly be rejected" (p. 286).

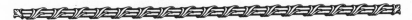

3

Working in Applied
Social Research:
A Selective Sample
of People and Projects

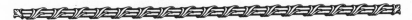

The previous chapter dealt with the intense experiences of four social science researchers outside the health services and gave some idea of the political atmosphere of applied social research in general. I turn now to some researchers who have worked mostly in the health field, and I present the range of their experiences, from the relatively noncontroversial to the controversial. Most of these researchers are sociologists, but two are economists, four are physicians as well as experts in management, and one is a physician who associates himself with sociology and political sociology. The researchers who have worked outside the health services have dealt with several problems: the recruiting of priests for the Catholic Church, the military establishment in the United States, and poverty and income redistribution. I do not claim that the researchers discussed here are statistically representative of health services researchers or researchers in other areas of social concern, but I believe that they do represent a range of experience in applied social research. I know them all personally; some are former students of mine. All cooperated enthusiastically.

Proper classification of problems in applied research is not easy to do. Some problems are not necessarily peculiar to applied research but are also inherent in theoretical research. In no particular order, these problems are the following:

- Access to research sites
- Availability of research funds, policies of funding agencies, and relationships with them

- Adequate time to carry out research (short-term versus long-term funding)
- The state of the art of methodology with respect to the practical problem being researched (Are there well-tested methodologies, or must one devise relatively new techniques?)
- Implementation of research findings that deal with administrators and policymakers
- Reporting style for disseminating results (scholarly or journalistic)
- Publication outlets and formats (books, monographs, articles)
- Cross-disciplinary cooperation in many applied research projects
- Role marginality in applied research
- Ideology and controversial social issues and interpretation
- Selection of research problems at any given time with respect to immediate or near-future policy relevance
- Appropriate timing of research results with respect to immediate policy relevance or relevance to the near future

Cecil G. Sheps

I shall start with the early researchers in what became known as health services research. One of them, Cecil G. Sheps, M.D., a Canadian, spent his early days in Saskatchewan. Before World War II, he was active in promoting medical care programs and health insurance in that province. Later, he became a leader in public health and health insurance on the North American continent, and he produced a great deal of relevant data related to those problems. He reported having had great difficulties with the medical profession in Saskatchewan at the time (telephone interview with author, October 11, 1989). He eventually moved to the United States and continued his activities in this country, with a great deal of success and general acceptance. He was executive director of the Beth Israel Hospital in Boston during the 1950s and conducted early internal research on case mix in the hospital, producing data that many found useful.

It is interesting that he had political difficulties in Saskatchewan, but not in the United States (although before he was offered the Beth Israel position, a prestigious post in hospital circles, his past activities were investigated; naturally, he had to pass muster with the medical profession in general and with the hospital's medical staff in particular). He was associated with the group-practice prepayment movement in the early days and with what became known as social medicine (the word *social* being associated with socialism at that time). He is probably best known as an academic physician, teaching and doing research in health services administration and public health problems. He is now Taylor Grandey Distinguished Professor of Social Medicine, Emeritus, University of North Carolina, and is still active. In the early days, he says, people pioneering in health services research had a mission; now it is only a job. I believe I shared his sense of mission.

I first got to know Sheps in the summer of 1951, when we each had a World Health Organization fellowship in social medicine in northern Europe. We were together in England and Sweden. In 1952, when I became research director of the Health Information Foundation and Sheps went to Beth Israel Hospital, I helped to subsidize some of his internal research. Sheps would not, I believe, regard himself as primarily a health services researcher; rather, he became known as a health policy analyst and policy promoter, one who used supporting facts. His publications along these lines of endeavor are extensive. His onetime research assistant, Mark G. Field, became a leading sociologist concerned with U.S.S.R. health services and promoted cross-national research.

Eli Ginzberg

Eli Ginzberg, an economist and professor emeritus from the School of Business, Columbia University, has been working with general manpower problems, as well as with health services. He has been a manpower consultant to Democratic and Republican administrations alike, from Eisenhower's on (Ginzberg, 1987, p. 66). He prides himself on his ability to straddle political parties. From 1941 to 1982, Ginzberg was continually in some kind of advisory position in Washington. He refers to two types of academics—outsiders and insiders—some of whom play both roles interchangeably. Ginzberg regards himself as a "perpetual" insider. He thought of himself as operating in the policy field the way a British civil servant does, giving advice—the same advice—to whatever party was in power. His research on manpower, hospital beds, the physician and nurse supply, and public-private interrelationships has been useful to the mainstream political forces in this country. Therefore, Ginzberg has not been embroiled in polarized controversies over public policy. This hardly means that he has not been forthright in his recommendations, however. In this connection, he is distressed by the gungho pace and pressures for change brought to bear on the traditional American delivery system—on voluntary hospitals and privately practicing physicians, with their time-honored responsibility to deliver high-quality medical care and to care for people who have no health insurance and otherwise fall between the cracks. In Ginzberg's view, the business-competition model is "destabilizing" an arrangement that was working reasonably well. He advises more effort to make the traditional system work in terms of cost containment, equity, and maintenance of quality (Ginzberg, 1989). He is trying to counter the forces of the business-competition model, which he sees as inappropriate to the health services. Even though he is an economist and supports a market economy, he believes that the health services are not a commodity but a public good.

Ginzberg sees himself as applying economics to policy problems; he does not pretend to subscribe to a particular macroeconomic theory. In his research reports, however, he implicitly and explicitly assumes a regulated laissez-faire capitalistic system, as well as the need for humane welfare-state capitalism. He has written many books and is in demand as a speaker adept at attacking policy illusions. Ginzberg's pragmatism is in the mold of the American political process. His positions fall within the American political tolerance range and combine goal advocacy with instrumental recommendations. He has many academic progeny.

Milton I. Roemer

Milton I. Roemer has been and continues to be the most prolific and wide-swinging health services researcher in the United States since the 1940s. I met him in 1943, when he was working for his M.P.H. (three years after earning his M.D.) at the School of

Public Health, University of Michigan. He came to study with Professor Nathan Sinai a year after I became Sinai's research assistant. Roemer and I were contemporaries, and we jokingly remarked that we did not know who was learning what from the other. In the 1930s, Roemer had intended to engage in community health work. Almost in passing, he picked up an M.A. in sociology from Cornell University before entering medical school at New York University.

Roemer was dedicated to applied research, in order to provide solid facts for policy papers. On occasion, he presented papers at conferences of sociologists, where he scolded his colleagues for engaging in "ivory tower" social research rather than attacking the festering problems of society, particularly in the health field. After some stints in public health service administration, he settled into a public health academic position at the University of California, Los Angeles.

In a memorandum to me about this book, Roemer revealed his faith in research to solve problems. He quoted his former classmate Jonas Salk, of polio vaccine fame: "If you ask the right question, nature never gives the wrong answer." Paraphrasing Salk, Roemer wrote: "I felt that one could substitute 'society' for 'nature' and the task was still to ask the right questions."

Roemer's first major opportunity to conduct applied research on his own terms came when he was in charge of the provincial hospital insurance program in Saskatchewan, from 1953 to 1956. Saskatchewan had established its insurance program in 1948. Roemer was struck and dismayed by the differences in rates of hospital use among the various areas of this rural prairie community of around a million people. What was causing these differences? Existing data, collected on hospitals for administrative purposes, could be analyzed. By picking the 50 localities with the highest hospitalization rates and the 50 with the lowest rates, out of a total of 360, Roemer found that in the high-hospitalization areas there tended to be a more rural population, low population density, and large families who lived greater distances from hospitals and had fewer physicians available. In the low-use-rate areas, he found the opposite characteristics.

In 1957, Roemer took a post in teaching and research at Cornell University. He learned of a Blue Cross plan in New York

State, where hospital costs were rising rapidly. The allegation was that the hospitals were being "overutilized." Roemer's answer, based on his Saskatchewan experience, was that the supply of hospital beds, the variable most subject to regulation, was associated with the alleged overuse. In fifty-six counties in New York State, and in the forty-seven other states, he found that about 70 percent of the variance in hospital admission rates could be attributed to the available bed supply. Hospitals were not any more crowded in the low-supply areas than in the high-supply areas. From this study emerged the generalization, an immediate classic, that "a bed built is a bed filled." It became known as Roemer's Law. This generalization was entered into testimony before a New York State legislative committee in December 1959. After five years of debate, New York State enacted legislation stipulating that no hospital could be enlarged or built without proof of the need for such action.

Roemer's research on hospital admission rates demonstrates his contention that socially useful research can be carried out at low cost. The data were already there, and permission was not needed to use them. The method was simple, the questions were relevant, and the policy implications were clear. Some researchers, however, would view this type of research as atheoretical; the generalizations are supposed to be self-evident.

In the mid 1960s, Roemer embarked on another research project, with colleagues from various disciplines and with data from agencies that had a vested interest in the results. In the United States, diverse health care delivery systems are owned by diverse entities, which claim to offer certain advantages for efficiency, health enhancement, and convenience. Three types of delivery systems that Roemer studied, this time in southern California, were the provider-sponsored Blue Cross and Blue Shield plans, private for-profit insurance plans, and group-practice prepayment plans. Among these three types of plans, what differences were there in use of services, costs, and attitudes of patients? The questions were simple enough, but the complexity and magnitude of the research methods were great.

A great deal of primary data needed to be collected, data that were not routinely available. Carefully randomized samples had to be selected from the total memberships of six health insurance organizations—two examples of each of the three types. Reliable statistics required sixty family units from each plan. This elaborate information had to be solicited, and privacy and confidentiality had to be respected. The project cost $1 million and involved twelve researchers over six years. When the study was well under way, according to Roemer, Blue Cross and Blue Shield, after extended and encouraging negotiations, decided not to participate, for reasons not mentioned. (I infer that so-called trade secrets were involved. Comparisons were not in the Blues' interests. Moreover, as is sometimes the case, there may have been distrust of the "liberal" tendencies of academic social science researchers.) The researchers then used a back-door strategy for obtaining samples of Blue Cross and Blue Shield members. They used a business directory of the local chamber of commerce to locate and consult several local labor unions, which had data on union members enrolled in the Blue plans.

Internal staff problems surfaced, not surprisingly for a project of this size. Some personality clashes probably had their origins in the arcane (from the lay standpoint) conceptual and methodological styles of the several disciplines engaged. This is a familiar problem of cross-disciplinary research, where everyone is supposed to be equal but some are more equal than others, not to mention more aggressive. It was legally necessary to obtain the cooperation of the physicians whose patients were being queried. Probably the stickiest problem was differences in interpreting results—"the subject of long debates," as Roemer put it. Nevertheless, these problems were overcome. The stakes were high, but the methodology passed muster in the health services research community, and trustworthy findings resulted from this large-scale pioneering study.

In June 1972, Roemer testified before a U.S. Senate subcommittee investigating monopolistic practices in the insurance industry. He presented the major comparative findings. The performance of the for-profit private insurance companies and the provider-sponsored plans was quite similar, in most respects. The insurance plan with "exceptional performance" was the one associated with the prepaid group-practice clinics in that their hospital-use rates were lower, there was greater contact with physicians, use of preventive services was higher, and expenditures per enrollee were lower (but not spectacularly so—$364 for the insurance and Blue plans versus $323 for the group-practice clinics). The proportion of enrollees dissatisfied with the medical care they received and with their degree of financial protection was significantly lower for the group-practice clinics than for the insurance and Blue plans (although such enrollees were a rather small minority in both instances).

Roemer and his associates received a lot of publicity for their testimony, and this is not surprising. In the 1960s, debates were intense on the advantages of the group-practice plans over mainstream insurance. There were few data of the kind reported by Roemer to show any comparisons. Roemer believes, plausibly enough, that his testimony may have had some influence on Congress's deliberations. The following year, Congress enacted legislation to subsidize start-up costs for such prepaid group-practice plans, which then became known as health-maintenance organizations (HMOs). The intention was to give HMOs a start by providing grants for capital. Later, the HMOs were to be on their own, competing with mainstream insurance plans in a clear example of public- and private-sector interrelationship. This concept did not sit well with the American Medical Association, however, for private physicians had to raise their own capital for their practices.

Roemer observed "many examples of difficulties and adjustments" with health services research in the United States, but his experiences with studies of health systems in other countries were "largely peaceful and positive." He is best known for his extensive cross-national investigations, but he denies that his international work was actual research, in the usual sense of the term (implying quasi-experimental, systematic surveys, and so on). Rather, he was called on by a number of countries (usually developing nations) and by the World Health Organization to describe and analyze health systems by using existing data and official reports and interviews. In a matter of weeks, he was to make recommendations to the governments that had requested this consultation. Roemer has covered over sixty countries, including industrialized nations. He has the intuitive capacity to cover more ground in less time, and to come up with more plausible observations, than anyone else in the field of health systems analysis. He would also be the first to say that a great deal more primary research must be done, beyond his own type of methodology, to foster understanding of the many "black boxes" of internal decision making. With all due respect to Roemer, I see him as largely an a priori analyst, with a model in his head for the proper organization and financing of health care delivery systems from country to country. It is the standard public health model of government funding through taxes, a great deal of structuring through regionalization, and more or less directed planning. This approach, of course, is congenial to developing countries, where government is perforce a leading change agent. Roemer reports having been quite successful in getting things started in various countries, El Salvador and Sri Lanka (then Ceylon) among others. He also set up "health demonstration areas" in some countries, as models for application.

One of Roemer's more interesting and amusing experiences was in 1979 in Barbados, an island state of 260,000 people. He was then being sponsored by the Inter-American Development Bank for a project that called for what the Barbados government named a National Health Service (in imitation of the former mother country). With a small group of colleagues from the Kaiser Foundation International, Roemer was put in charge of working out Phase I, a program of primary health care for everyone on the island. It was very difficult to gather information on all forms of primary health care, particularly from private general practitioners. It was difficult even to get answers to simple questions, such as how many physicians in active practice were generalists and how many specialists. There was a policy agreement that financing would be mainly through incremental contributions from the social insurance fund for old-age pensions, which had been in operation for some years. No one knew, however, how many dependents were linked to each primary worker, and it was important to know how many people could be financed through social insurance. Therefore, field surveys became necessary. It was learned eventually that insured persons plus dependents would account for 82 percent of the island population; thus, only 18 percent of the population needed to be financed from general revenues. The latter source raises, of course, the sticky political issue of personal progressive income taxes. A less simply mechanical problem of data collection was encountered: to determine the income of private general practitioners, the researchers wanted to look into confidential income records by examining income tax returns. This proposal was flatly rejected, even when it was emphasized that no names were needed. When it occurred to Roemer that the research project, "without implying bribery," could pay double for the overtime work that the estimates would require, the figures were produced in a few days.

The Barbados government was pleased with the research team's proposals, including the one for cost estimates. The researchers made a request to meet with the Barbados Medical Association for a general discussion of the plan. The association held off until the last night of Roemer's stay. Roemer reports, "The initial reception to my talk was polite, if rather quiet, but then the fireworks began. The opposition, it turned out, came not from the general practitioners, but from the specialists. Organizations of seventy primary-care teams [these were what was recommended] would suddenly deprive these specialists—who were supposedly on full-time salaries in the single large hospital on the island—of their private patients seen in the evenings." The opposition of the specialists was neutralized when the government was persuaded to increase their salaries. This did take some time.

By this time, however, some general practitioners began to fear the specter of excessive government intervention in medical practice. An election was coming up, and the cabinet was pushed into a decision to postpone final action until after the election. Roemer reports that by 1985 no action on social insurance to support primary health care had yet been taken. The government was still in favor of the idea, but the time was not "politically ripe." What Roemer and others have discovered, of course, is that in countries with independent medical practitioners (or even practitioners who are not so independent), the medical profession has to be accommodated in one way or another.

As Roemer concludes his memorandum to me, "Above all, in my view, is the importance of my opening remark about asking the right questions. If one has some sociological imagination, it is often possible to make use of *already existing data* [emphasis in the original] to answer questions that are crucial to public policy decisions.

Even if the answers are not immediately translatable into social actions, they can point decision makers in the right direction."

What Roemer points out is that discipline-oriented researchers need to be more problem-oriented in health services research in order to be useful to policy formulation. This continues to be a basic dilemma for academically based researchers. Policy-oriented research needs to continue to be "mission"-oriented, as Cecil G. Sheps has observed. Roemer represents an endangered species in that few researchers are still willing to express strong advocacy on the basis of research results. Roemer, by being a sophisticated polemicist and drawing on supportive data, quite gracefully survived the slings and arrows of his advocacy for drastic reorganization and funding for the health services.

Ronald Andersen

Ronald Andersen can be regarded as a second-generation health services researcher and medical sociologist. I hired him in 1963, a year after the Health Information Foundation and my staff moved to the Graduate School of Business at the University of Chicago. Andersen had completed his Ph.D. examinations in sociology at Purdue University and was looking for a topic and data for his dissertation. I was looking for someone to be the project director for my third nationwide household survey on use of and expenditures for personal health services. As before, I contracted with the National Opinion Research Center to conduct the survey portion of the study and produce the desired data. I began as the principal investigator, but after watching Andersen take hold during the first six months of the survey's formulation and staging, I suggested that he be the principal investigator and that I be the junior author. (By this time, I had become punch-drunk fielding nationwide surveys and was glad to place the major logistical burden on someone else I trusted.) Andersen was primarily responsible for writing the report of this survey. From it, he produced his dissertation (Andersen, 1968), which has become a reference model for the study of access to health services.

Andersen's research was not controversial until he and his associates began to probe the impact of the Reagan administration's policies on the Medicaid program. The Robert Wood Johnson Foundation wished to learn what the effects were of Reagan's fiscal and eligibility restrictions on access to care for Medicaid recipients and those immediately above the official poverty level (interview with author, December 15, 1988). There were two surveys, one in 1982 and the other in 1986. With respect to the 1982 survey, to paraphrase Andersen, the proponents of greater equity and access to services were critical of its methodology, saying it was not sensitive to the nuances of the inequity between the poor and the well-off; they did not believe that the partial convergence, over time, of access for the poor and the well-off was as great as the survey showed. The "conservatives," however, took heart that things were not as bad as the "liberals" claimed. The Robert Wood Johnson Foundation was also concerned but published the findings (the foundation was already committed to having the results published by one means or another). Andersen himself was surprised by the findings because he had intuitively expected a wider difference. The critics claimed that the poor are less aware of their needs than are the well-off who have Medicaid insurance, and that the concept of need among the poor should be brought on a par with that of the well-off; the perceived needs of the well-off are greater than their objective needs and result in this group's overuse of services.

The results of the 1986 survey did show decline in access for the poor and the uninsured; but, again, it was hardly a pronounced decline, according to Andersen. Once again, the critics believed that the level of access for the poor was worse than the data showed, because the indicators were not sensitive enough. One explanation, according to Andersen, is that it takes more than four years to see the full impact of reduced financing in Medicaid programs and to see an increase in the uninsured population on the basis of access levels.

What is worse or better is, of course, a matter of definitions (which actors on each side of an issue carry in their heads for purposes of political action). The liberals look for the worst data, the conservatives for the best. Andersen is very conscious of the policy implications of his research; indeed, his choice of problems for research shows that awareness. At the same time, he is very careful to see that his methodology is sound. Even so, he inevitably gets caught in the crossfire.

A broader problem, which has confronted Andersen with increasing intensity, is support from the University of Chicago Graduate School of Business. The research problems that Andersen believes are pertinent to the health field are peripheral to the heavy emphasis on economics at the University of Chicago, with respect to research as well as to courses offered in the Center for Health Administration Studies within the Graduate Program in Health Administration (Andersen is director of both). Four successive deans between 1962 and 1984 were very supportive of the center's and the program's activities. In 1984, however, the support of the dean's office became tenuous, for two major reasons. One was the tightening of academic resources after a long period of affluence. The other concerned the fact that the Graduate Program in Health Administration was the only industry-specific program in the Graduate School of Business. It was the only one of its type to be retained after the school's quite thorough restructuring of its curriculum, in the early 1960s. The philosophy of the Graduate School of Business was that a University of Chicago M.B.A., given the process and management philosophy to which the students were exposed, was trained to run any enterprise. Hence, health administration was an anomaly in the school. (In effect, Andersen also became an anomaly, given his competence and interests, although his tenure was not in question; there are behavioral scientists on the faculty who are working on organization and decision making.) In any case, the program, founded in 1934, had attained a national and international reputation that was helped considerably by its being situated within the Graduate School of Business, with its stellar faculty in finance, marketing, accounting, and so on. Essentially, however, with a new dean and scarce support from the general faculty, the program as such has been abolished, and only a core of health care-related courses are being retained.

The Center for Health Administration Studies recently underwent scrutiny by a university committee with respect to its seating and to space for it elsewhere in the university. It was decided to seat it within the School of Social Service Administration. There will be four tracks for health services administration: the School of

Social Service Administration, the School of Policy, the School of Business, and the Division of Biological Sciences. There is cross-department and cross-school interest, from social work to medicine; the center has always been host to cross-disciplinary research and teaching. Given the serious and massive problems of the health field today, which cut across so many interests within the university, the attempt is to create a universitywide arrangement, with the new Graduate School of Policy Studies, the School of Social Service Administration, and the Graduate School of Business all under a supervisory committee.

It is apparent that in the health field and in its teaching and research, there are external as well as internal political problems and issues. Externally, the problems are politically controversial. Internally, the problems are departmental, disciplinary, and school-related. The health services field falls between academic stools everywhere, no matter where it is seated—in schools of public health, schools of management, or medical schools. In other words, Andersen has been caught in a problem of structure, a problem largely independent of him as a scholar.

Gretchen Voorhis Fleming

Gretchen Voorhis Fleming was on the staff of the Center for Health Administration Studies at the University of Chicago when I was director. She earned her Ph.D. in sociology at the University of Chicago, and I was on her dissertation committee. She eventually became research director at the American Academy of Pediatrics.

Her experience with her dissertation is of interest here because she got so far into the complexities of various levels of authority that her proposal appeared to have been accepted at all levels but was finally rejected at the top level of the department involved (personal correspondence, January 5, 1989). She formulated a project in the early 1970s to study the development of the role of the nurse-midwife in the prenatal and obstetrical units run by the Department of Obstetrics and Gynecology in a large hospital in Chicago. Her entreé was the head of the Department of Maternal and Child Nursing of a nearby university, who had contacts with the hospital. I wrote a supporting letter. Fleming's proposal, referred to a high official in the hospital for approval, also had to involve the Scientific Committee on Human Experimentation. From there, the proposal—supported so far—was submitted to the head of the Department of Obstetrics and Gynecology, who approved it. This process took from April to June 1973 to complete. From there, the process slowed down considerably as questions were raised about methodology, and it was suggested that there be a coinvestigator from the hospital.

From June 1973, after the director of the Department of Obstetrics and Gynecology had approved the proposal, until April 23, 1974, almost a year later, the proposal was in a "black box" of internal ambivalence about whether to accept the proposal. On April 23, Fleming received a letter dated March 26 but postmarked April 22, announcing that her project had been rejected.

What Fleming learned from this experience is that a researcher should not undertake a project when the following three conditions exist: (1) the researcher does not know the politics of the institution involved, nor does the researcher have a disinterested informant; (2) the researcher is an outsider; and (3) the researcher is asked to submit the project more than twice to the same or new bodies.

Grace Budrys

Grace Budrys earned her Ph.D. in sociology at the University of Chicago in 1976. I was the chair of her dissertation committee. She is now professor of sociology and director of the Public Service Program at De Paul University, Chicago.

As part of her research endeavors at De Paul University, she became interested in studying how the Chicago Health Service Agency (HSA), one of the local agencies of the National Health Services Planning Act of 1974, was responding to the cutting off of federal funds by the Reagan administration in 1982. What does an institution do when it is doomed to die for lack of funds (personal correspondence, December 8, 1988)?

Budrys wrote to the director of HSA and asked permission to examine records that had accumulated since 1974 and to study the operation of the agency over the previous year. The response was that the files were open to anyone who was interested. In due course, she found out that the rich data files she had envisioned either did not exist or were too disorderly to be of much use. (Incidentally, this is a common experience of researchers who wish to delve into the records of agencies.) Budrys then resorted mainly to passive observation, by attending board meetings for many months and interviewing many informants.

She strategically presented two options of approach to the agency. One was to study the organizational response to a cut in funding (an approach implying, of course, a dying agency). The other approach was to study what the agency had achieved during its lifetime. After reviewing the letter in which Budrys outlined these two approaches, the assistant director of the agency invited Budrys for an interview. No interest at all was shown in the first option, but there was strong interest, understandably, in studying the achievements of the agency. Within a month of the executive committee's favorable vote, Budrys was able to start her study.

The day Budrys arrived to begin her study, she was introduced to the staff, and one member was assigned the task of getting her acquainted with the organization. Since there were many committees and a broad range of people from a cross-section of society, Budrys had some problems (none serious) explaining her role. Was she a student, an investigator, a reporter? Her detached research stance was not easy to explain.

Budrys reported to me that as she gained the trust of many agency people interviewed, she even got some voluntary "inside dope." When Budrys finished the report, she had become so enmeshed with the staff with whom she worked that she let some of them read the report. She hoped that they would think the report was fair; she knew they would not think it was flattering. Budrys was relieved that the readers did think the report was fair.

Merwyn R. Greenlick

For over twenty years, Merwyn R. Greenlick has been building up a health services research unit in a prominent HMO, Kaiser Permanente (Northwest Region, Portland, Oregon). The publication of a recent book by Greenlick and his associates, on the operation and accomplishments of this research unit, has made it easier to learn about the problems of health services research as associated with operating an HMO (personal interview at annual meeting of the Association of Health Services Research, Chicago, June 1989).

The development and strategy of the Center for Health Research, as the unit is now called, can be used as a case study of how an ongoing program of research attached itself to the HMO of which it both is and is not a part. The concept of a research unit at the Kaiser Permanente facility was conceived as early as 1959 by Ernest W. Saward, M.D., the Kaiser Northwest Region's founding medical director. The several Kaiser Permanente regions on the West Coast could decide for themselves how to spend the budgets allotted to them for a program of "education, research, and charitable care" (Greenlick, Freeborn, and Pope, 1988, p. 15). Other regions dedicated their funds to basic biomedical-clinical research, or to studying medical methods (a bioengineering approach to research). Saward, however, perceived the program as a significant social experiment that should be "seriously introspective." The program should develop a health services research laboratory to provide data for the field in general.

Greenlick was engaged to head this research unit in 1964. He had been trained in research and medical care organization in the School of Public Health at the University of Michigan (a unit I had helped Nathan Sinai to establish in 1945).

According to Greenlick, the organizational characteristics of an HMO are hospitable to health services research. An HMO has an identified and relatively stable population base. There is access to an integrated health care system, which has a stake in solving health services problems. There is also readily accessible and complete medical information on each individual in the population at risk, in one record, as well as information about types of patient-staff encounters, diagnosis, treatment modalities, and so on.

An initial and critical decision was whether the research program would become a research-and-development arm of the HMO administration (a staff function) or orient itself toward research that could be generalized to health services operations in the public domain (the HMO as a research laboratory). Portland Kaiser decided to do both, with funding from the HMO and from outside sources.

The research staff is intellectually independent of Kaiser Permanente's administrative structure, although the research director reports to top management as a vice-president. The Center for Health Research is in a separate facility from the HMO and has developed its own staff. This is a structural strategy intended to avoid the natural tendency "for researchers, who are HMO employees, to take on the values and norms and to behave as conforming members of the specific organization rather than as objective observers and researchers" (Greenlick, Freeborn, and Pope, 1988, p. 21). Another balancing act involves the staff. It is organized on a collegial model, to ensure staff members' independence and scientific integrity. Nevertheless, it is not "merely an umbrella for totally independent researchers selecting their own topics as their interests or the availability of support funds move[s] them" (Greenlick, Freeborn, and Pope, 1988, p. 23). Still, in the care and feeding of staff, so to speak, "the ability to work in an environment that supports academic values and permits the professional to achieve a successful career is a crucial element in sustaining the motivation and the commitment of research personnel" (Greenlick, Freeborn, and Pope, 1988, p. 26).

Although a unit like the Center for Health Research is closely related to the operational problems of an HMO, there still has to be diplomacy in getting access to the records of patients and their physicians. Health personnel are sensitive to research interventions and have to be persuaded that the research is worth their time and the intrusion; "they will, therefore, calculate their own cost-benefit ratios comparing the costs to themselves, as individuals, with whatever benefits they can see might derive from research outcomes. That assessment is likely to make some individuals in crucial positions cool to specific research projects" (Greenlick, Freeborn, and Pope, 1988, p. 28).

I asked Greenlick if there had been any major difficulties with the health personnel over research interventions, and he reported that there had been, but only twice in over twenty years. A perusal of the projects and their results makes it apparent that the Center for Health Research has been eminently successful in carrying out its mission by combining research relevant to the needs of Kaiser Permanente as well as to the general health field.

Jack Elinson

Jack Elinson's career is of interest here because he brought a background in social psychology to health services research. He got his start by doing research for the military during World War II (with the Samuel Stouffer research branch of *American Soldier* fame). Elinson reports that in the military, health and health services were not considered as sociologically interesting as race relations, relations between officers and enlisted men, reasons why we were fighting, draftees' morale, and other subjects (memoranda of August 10, 1988, and November 29, 1989; letter to author, October 3, 1988; telephone interview with author, October 21, 1988). Because medical care was highly regarded by servicemen, it was not a problem, and so it had a low sociological priority. Elinson says, modestly, that in these circumstances health services were not assigned to the best sociological analysts from high-prestige departments of sociology (an exception involved research on psychiatric screening, which turned out to make methodological as well as substantive contributions).

Elinson says that he was a sociologically untrained person, low on the totem pole. He was assigned to do research on morale in military hospitals and on prevention of trench foot. (Only later did he learn that his work on trench foot was called *epidemiology.*) He says that this experience was a piece of luck, because later on the National Opinion Research Center, with which he was affiliated in 1951, needed someone to work on its Commission on Chronic Illness. (Elinson also became associated with the national household survey that formed part of a study I conducted for the National Opinion Research Center.)

The Commission on Chronic Illness, sponsored by philanthropic foundations, was in Chicago at that time, over forty years ago. It was a pioneering attempt to explore empirically the dimensions of long-term illness. The prevailing emphasis on acute illness needed to be expanded to include chronic illness as an emerging and massive health problem, associated mostly with increasing length of life. The commission also intended to explore the question of preventing chronic illness early in the life span. The director of the commission, Morton Levin, M.D., was unable to raise enough money to do the kind of elaborate, national epidemiological study he felt was needed. The compromise was to do one rural and one urban survey. Levin resigned as director, for reasons unknown to Elinson, and was replaced by Dean Roberts, M.D., of Johns Hopkins University's School of Hygiene. Roberts accepted the appointment on the condition that the commission's headquarters be moved to Baltimore and that the urban component of the chronic-illness studies be carried out there. As for the rural study, Ray Trussell, M.D., who elsewhere had been a colleague of Levin's, had recently become director of what was to be the first medical center in Hunterdon County, New Jersey, and convinced the commission that Hunterdon County would be an appropriate site for the rural study. (This was before construction of the Hunterdon Medical Center, which was to combine personal and public health services.)

The biggest problem that the commission faced in its research was a methodological one: the categories *rural* and *urban* were rather general variables. Moreover, the question of how to define chronic illness and elicit data on it from a population represented pioneering research. Elinson says that, after the results from Hunterdon County became known, he went through an "inquisition" by statisticians in the relevant department of the federal government. This was happening just before the National Center for Health Statistics was established. A major question that the National Center for Health Statistics was facing—one with which Elinson and the Commission on Chronic Illness were also coming to grips in their pioneering research—was how to go about doing surveys to assess the nation's health. From this experience was formulated the Health Examination Survey, which became an important source of data on the nation's health.

Elinson went on to become a professor in Columbia University's School of Public Health and Administrative Medicine, where Ray Trussell was dean, and became a leading contributor to social epidemiology until his retirement, several years ago; it appears that his research on trench foot was indeed an appropriate springboard for his career. I asked Elinson if he had felt marginal as a sociologist in a biologically oriented academic environment. He replied that he had always felt marginal but used his marginality creatively.

Sol Levine

Sol Levine was another early entrant into health services research. He joined my research staff at the Health Information Foundation in 1954, to head a project on the problems that Blue Cross plans had in enrolling self-employed people. Levine had just earned his Ph.D. in sociology from New York University and was oriented toward both applied research and sociological theory.

He kindly told me that, by working with me, he learned a great deal of social research strategy—for example, to use the right euphemisms in speaking with sensitive agencies (*private insurance* rather than *commercial insurance*) (telephone interview with author, October 31, 1988). The Blue Cross plans did not want to be associated with the term *insurance* at all; they preferred *prepayment*. This was at a time when there was intense competition between the Blue Cross–Blue Shield plans and the private insurance companies (technically known as *stock companies*). The Blue plans wanted the image of a nonprofit organization in the context of health insurance and health services. The intensity of the "battle of designations" in the 1950s would be hard to overstate.

Levine went on to the Russell Sage Foundation, as a fellow in medical sociology. After stints at Harvard's School of Public Health and Johns Hopkins University's School of Hygiene, he became a professor in the Department of Sociology at Boston University, where he has been for some years. He was recently on leave, to serve as vice-president for program development at the Kaiser Family Foundation in California, but at this writing he is back in Boston.

Levine's major work has probably been in the social psychology of coping with chronic illness, such as heart disease and cancer. For example, a pharmaceutical company financed a study that Levine and his colleagues carried out on the differential effects of three major antihypertensive medications on patients' quality of life (Croog and others, 1986). The researchers found that different drugs did indeed have different effects on quality of life, effects that could be gauged with psychosocial measures. In such research, Levine has naturally dealt with distress on the part of drug firms hoping for different results.

Morris Janowitz

The late Morris Janowitz and I were colleagues at the University of Chicago's Department of Sociology. Thus, in addition to the works I cite, I can also draw on my occasional interchanges with him from 1962 to 1988. Janowitz is best known, both within and outside sociology, for his work on the military establishment of the United States.

In an interview with Bernard Barber, Janowitz explained how he became the macrosociologist he was and selected the sociological problems he did. His mother, an Eastern European Jewish immigrant, made him very aware of the political unrest and change in Europe. That awareness, he said in the interview, made him "wary of broad social movements and efforts toward wholesale social change" (Janowitz, 1987, p. 66). His wariness is revealed in his work on institution building and social change. Janowitz believed that in the organization of research there should be sharp differentiation between applied and basic research. The greater the differentiation, he believed, the less effective one's work in influencing policy.

With respect to the military establishment, his specific policy goals were not only to increase the public's knowledge of the military but also to increase the military's knowledge of itself. (In fact, the military establishment purchased thousands of copies of his book *The Professional Soldier,* published in 1960 and revised in 1965.) Janowitz did not accept money from the Department of Defense (which he apparently could have done), for strategic reasons: aside from the issue of so-called tainted money, he thought his students would object. He also observed that most sociologists think it is morally wrong to study the military, because such attention seems to imply that the military is an acceptable social institution.

Janowitz saw a fundamental tension between the professional soldier and the scholar, with the latter seeking to apply the methods of social science to a study of the human side of military organization and armed conflict. The professional soldier often sees the social scientist as naïve but must defer to him or her out of professional courtesy because the scholar has permission to study him. On the other side, the social scientist views the professional soldier as dogmatic. Until Janowitz (1965), the approach of social scientists to the military establishment was segmental and technical, rather than comprehensive and scientific.

Janowitz constructed new ways of stating old problems. For example, he formulated the concepts of the citizen-soldier and of constabulary functions to maintain the peace (as well as offensive and defensive functions). From his study of the military, he learned that sociologists had to be staff rather than line professionals (Barber, 1987, p. 75). In his view, sociology can help clarify the questions that people have to decide on and answer, but it cannot answer specific questions. Janowitz chose the Enlightenment model for social science, not the engineering model characteristic of the physical sciences. He liked to emphasize the voluntarism of social action and decision making and disliked what he regarded as the rigid determinism of some economic and sociological models. His work on the military and its personnel problems teaches that it is not easy to effect lasting social change, certainly not in the short run.

Norman Gevitz

Norman Gevitz earned his Ph.D. in sociology at the University of Chicago in 1980. I was the chairman of his dissertation committee. His dissertation was a definitive study of the development of osteopathic medicine as an institution in the United States. Given the traditional marginality of osteopathy (at least until recently) and its struggle to gain medical respectability, Gevitz was concerned with getting access to osteopaths (D.O.s) and freedom to publish his results. He was interested in occupational role duplication in medicine, specifically where such fields as dentistry, podiatry, and optometry overlapped with mainstream medicine in scope of practice. By reviewing the literature, he learned that very little had been written about osteopathic medicine, but D.O.s were licensed in all fifty states and in the District of Columbia, separately from M.Ds.

Gevitz learned that there was a school of osteopathic medicine only a few blocks from the University of Chicago. He knew no one in osteopathic medicine, and so he took the unusual first step of writing directly to George Northup, D.O., editor of various

American Osteopathic Association (AOA) publications, to an-
nounce his interest and request a meeting (personal correspondence,
December 5, 1988). Northup's reply was most cordial, and Gevitz
was referred to the executive director of the AOA, Edward Crowell,
D.O. Northup also sent copies of Gevitz's letter to other colleagues,
which made Gevitz fear that access to information "might involve
a group decision, and layers of bureaucracy." This fear proved
groundless, however. Gevitz met with Crowell and explained what
he wanted to do (at that time it was called *historical sociology;* later
it came to be called *social history*). He told Crowell that the study
would be a scholarly one; its value to the profession would be self-
knowledge. Crowell's response was enthusiastic. He promised to
make all records available and provide working space. He also said
that he wanted no control over the content of the study.

Crowell also described a previous experience with a study of
osteopathic medicine. An employee of the AOA was commissioned
by the association to write a popular history of the profession, and
a contract was signed with a major publisher. This book was
stopped after an "oversight committee" objected to the content of
some early chapters. When the author refused to make changes, the
agreement with the author was rescinded, as was the contract with
the publisher. Crowell did not want this experience repeated, and
he instructed all relevant departments of the AOA headquarters to
cooperate with Gevitz. All of them did. Gevitz believes that Crowell
offered "protection" (if that was needed). It was also his impression
that members of the board of trustees and the house of delegates,
when they came to the Chicago headquarters, did not know who he
was and what he was doing: publicity might have raised awkward
questions. Gevitz kept a low profile. His research was based more
on library and archival materials than on interviews. He says he
maintained a "shadow presence."

The timing of the project was nearly perfect. The osteopathic
profession had just won some key legislative victories. The profession, after a period of much internal questioning about its survival,
was on the upswing. Several new schools were started, a number of
them affiliated with universities. What the profession suffered from
was social invisibility in that most people had only a vague understanding, or none at all, of osteopathic medicine. Perhaps, Gevitz

thought, whatever he wrote in his book would give the profession greater visibility. If he provided straightforward information about what D.O.s did, the traditional stereotypes would yield to a more positive image. Gevitz believes that Crowell also recognized this possibility: "In this case I believe it was not so much my developing a good strategy to get cooperation . . . as it was the preexisting attitude of the principal individual I was to deal with and the . . . favorable timing of my project and what . . . potential positive effects it was perceived it could produce." The book (Gevitz, 1982) was published by Johns Hopkins University Press and was well received by osteopaths.

John E. Kralewski

John E. Kralewski is professor and director of the Division of Health Services Research and Policy, School of Public Health, at the University of Minnesota, Minneapolis. He sees his main problems as the administration of a research establishment and the gaining of access to what are viewed as sensitive data.

In a letter and an interview, Kralewski lists three problems (telephone interview with author, October 17, 1988; personal correspondence, December 22, 1988). The first centers on the difficulties associated with developing a sustained research effort, focused on a specific problem, that can make a real contribution in the long run. Funding sources and their expectations are problematic; this research unit is quite closely related to the needs and problems of the state of Minnesota, an arrangement that implies short-term funding and fast production. Kralewski also feels that the natural tendencies of discipline-trained investigators to focus on theory and methods, rather than on practical problems, is a problem in health services research. Kralewski is very problem- and policy-oriented. He wants to solve health problems and improve administration, and he feels the lack of similarly oriented researchers.

The second problem, somewhat related to the first, is getting interdisciplinary teams to work effectively together. Most problems in health services research do require interdisciplinary teams.

The third problem is obtaining data from health care providers as the field becomes increasingly competitive. Many of today's important issues in health care delivery require data from providers who are reluctant to share information. Data collection has become somewhat easier, however, as organizations (hospital systems, group practices, and so on) have become larger. Nevertheless, there is a real "source of data" issue. Kralewski said that physicians in Hennepin County, which includes Minneapolis, are concerned about falling income and the erosion of health care's quality but are reluctant to finance or invite research on these important problems.

Richard Shoenherr

Richard Shoenherr is professor of sociology at the University of Wisconsin–Madison. His major interest is the sociology of religion. For fifteen years, he has been studying problems in recruiting priests for the Catholic Church in the United States (personal interviews, October 24, 1988, and November 17, 1989). He has the backing of the top hierarchy of the church, who sought the study because of their concern about the dwindling supply of priests. Shoenherr's project studies demographic changes in the priesthood, as well as priests' attitudes toward celibacy and the traditional role demands of the church. An early phase of the study was funded, to the tune of $300,000, by the United States Catholic Conference. The later phase was funded by the Lilly Foundation and sponsored by the conference. Funding was shifted to the foundation because the conference was distressed by what was bad news, from its perspective: that priests had critical attitudes toward celibacy and the pope.

One of the study's basic methods was to mail a questionnaire to seven thousand priests. Five thousand questionnaires were returned. In the next stage of the project, Shoenherr constructed a census of the clergy and made population projections to the year 2005.

The bishop of the conference approved the instrument question by question, with respect to how moral and theological elements were handled. The demographic techniques were also given official approval. Since the study had the approval of the conference, bishops in individual dioceses were less reluctant to release sensitive personnel data (about resignations, for example). Within the rest of the Catholic hierarchy, there were mixed responses, although there was enough support in principle to keep the project going. The hierarchy wanted the research information for internal policy purposes, and it preferred sponsoring an independent project to diverting money from its central missions and doing the research itself.

An interesting and significant feature of this research, given its subject matter and the institution being studied, is that its results will be published. After reviewing the early data, the bishops raised the question of control and ownership of the data: Couldn't the report just be shoved under a desk? They called in legal counsel and were advised that the conference, having contracted for a study with a professional sociologist from a well-recognized university, must therefore respect the academic researcher's professional norms and standards. There the matter rests. A publisher has already been found. After publication, the church, like any other critic, can attack the study if it wants to.

The study is taking a long time because of slow decision-making clearance within the church hierarchy. Shoenherr, a practicing Catholic, is also a former priest, married to a former nun, and his directing a project like this one was seen as somewhat questionable. Since the study involves an unusual combination of sensitive issues—celibacy, sexuality, theology, the shortage of priests, church governance—it seems that this project is as deep a probing into the "black boxes" of a complex organization as has ever been carried out. There is no direct censorship. It is not an in-house study of the kind usually carried out by institutions. Shoenherr reports that there is intense interest in this study, mainly because of the shortage of priests. He gets telephone calls weekly from people in the news media. He plans a well-managed press conference for disclosing the study's results, so that he can control interpretation of the data as much as possible, control being a constant problem in relationships between social scientists and the news media.

Stephen M. Shortell

Data may throw a public policy, particularly one that concerns life and death, into question. This fact was illustrated by Stephen M. Shortell and Edward F. X. Hughes in an article that appeared in the *New England Journal of Medicine* (Shortell and Hughes, 1988). Shortell says that the Health Care Finance Administration (HCFA) was quite distressed by the article, which reports the results of a study that examined how the regulation of hospital rates, state certificate-of-need programs, competition, and hospital ownership affected mortality rates among inpatients receiving Medicare-funded treatment for sixteen selected conditions. Data were obtained from the records of 214,839 inpatients in 981 hospitals in forty-five states, from July 1, 1983, through June 30, 1984. The news that upset HCFA was that the authors had found significant positive associations between higher inpatient mortality, on the one hand, and, on the other, the stringency of state programs for reviewing hospital rates, the stringency of certificate-of-need legislation, and the intensity of competition (as measured by enrollment in HMOs). Hospitals in the states that had the most stringent rate-review procedures had death rates 6 to 10 percent higher than the death rates of hospitals in states with less stringent rate-review procedures. Similar differences, of varying degrees, were found for the other variables. Naturally, these findings raised serious concerns about the welfare of patients admitted to hospitals in highly regulated areas and in relatively competitive markets. It thus became apparent that it is important to use quality-assurance procedures and systems to monitor outcomes. According to Shortell, HCFA took three staff members off regular duty in the Baltimore office to replicate the data (personal interview, November 17, 1988). Many newspapers ran stories on this article, and the authors had many telephone calls, all very time-consuming.

I asked Shortell how he defines himself. He said that he is an organizational theorist. When he was a student in the University of Chicago's Graduate School of Business, earning a Ph.D. in behavioral sciences, he was based in the Center for Health Administration Studies, of which I was director. He is now a professor in the J. L. Kellogg Graduate School of Management at Northwestern University and is also associated with the Center for Health Services and Policy Research.

David Mechanic

David Mechanic became a major contributor to research in medical sociology in the 1950s, when he was in the Department of Sociology at the University of Wisconsin–Madison. In 1980, he moved to Rutgers University, where he has established a thriving center for health services research. His major interest has been the social psychological aspects of the health services, as well as their organization.

Mechanic reports that his biggest problem has been gaining access to data from big firms and their benefits managers on their experiences with benefit plans, HMOs, and other providers (telephone interview, October 10, 1988). The competitive environment has become so intense that the firms are reluctant to release data into the public domain, although they are avid for data in general. Firms' representatives also say that their employees, as a matter of privacy, may not want to be interviewed. At least in the earlier days, Blue Cross–Blue Shield plans appeared easier to gain access to. By the time of my interview with Mechanic, however, the business atmosphere had changed, and he has received many requests from HMOs for research on their experiences—but they are not willing to pay for the studies. Mechanic says that the best way to get access to data is to deal with strategically placed gatekeepers whom he already knows. Even they, however, are not enough to gain him entry, for the self-protective policies of the firms are enough to prevent it.

I asked Mechanic if he has felt marginal in the field of sociology, being a medical sociologist. He said that he had not, and that he sees himself as a sociologist who has an interest in medical sociology. He is now setting up an interdisciplinary research team because separate disciplines are too confining for his current research tasks.

Robert Lampman

Robert Lampman was my major informant on the establishment of the Institute for Research on Poverty, seated in the Department of Economics at the University of Wisconsin–Madison. As a professor of economics, Lampman specialized in social insurance and general public welfare. He retired in 1988 (personal interview, April 23, 1989).

The institute was established in 1966. It originated from the activities of the Council of Economic Advisers and the group of policy advisers assembled by the newly elected Johnson administration in 1964. The council was headed by the late Walter Heller of the University of Minnesota, who was regarded as a liberal economist. Lampman was a member of the council for two years.

According to Lampman, the institute received block grants to study what seemed important to the faculties in economics, social work, and sociology, within the general mission of understanding the phenomenon of poverty in an affluent society. The University of Wisconsin's administration was a bit hesitant to accept government money for so inherently political a mission. Likewise, some academic critics felt that the institute was too mission-oriented in that it seemed to be helping policymakers who were then in power by serving as their research agency. Presumably, individual faculty members, as free academicians, could serve the government as consultants (this was a very common and accepted practice), but the apparently "official" funding of the institute seemed worrisome.

In any case, according to Haveman (1987, p. 8), the institute was very prolific in its publications. Between 1965 and 1980, the institute published 35 books, 650 discussion papers, and 18 special reports. It spent $20 million, mostly from the federal government. It was a focal point for scholars, in several disciplines and from numerous universities and institutions, who were interested in poverty research and antipoverty policy. By the time the Reagan administration came into power, in 1981, the government's interest in research on poverty had weakened considerably, and the institute's appropriations were a casualty of the general retrenchment. According to Haveman, the funding provided to the institute had more influence on the direction of economists' research than it did on public policy.

Rockwell Schulz

Rockwell Schulz established the Program in Health Services Administration at the University of Wisconsin–Madison in the mid 1970s. It is based in the medical school's Department of Preventive Medicine and has tracks in that department, in industrial engineering, in the business school, and in policy and planning. His major interest is research in health services organization. As usual with an academic field that has no central discipline and is relatively new, the establishment of the Program in Health Services Administration entailed negotiations and bargaining.

According to Schulz, an important and persistent problem for health services researchers is differences in the data needs of managers, consultants, and researchers. Managers and consultants want rather specific data for specific decisions within an organization (personal interview, October 15, 1988). They are atheoretical and want facts for immediate decision making. Academically based researchers find it difficult to operate with such expectations. Research takes time and money, often beyond the resources and patience of the people who will use its results. Good evaluation is expensive.

Access to research sites also takes time to develop. Schulz cites his experience with cross-national research in mental health administration in the United Kingdom, West Germany, and the United States. Schulz tries to work with existing systems (such as trauma programs and HMOs) in his cross-national research. For example, he has found costs in private mental hospitals to be higher than in public hospitals, but this finding has caused no particular stir.

He has had some difficulty publishing his study of the HMOs in Dane County, Wisconsin, which contains the city of Madison. (There is a very high penetration of HMO competition in that area.) His findings were quite favorable on HMOs' popularity with members and the cooperation of physicians. Schulz says that the *Journal of the American Medical Association* rejected his article because it seemed biased toward the HMOs, according to the journal's reviewer. He finally did publish his study, however (Schulz, Girard, and Harrison, 1990).

Another problem that Schulz mentioned, which has become general among researchers, is the tremendous investment of time and the lead time necessary to formulate grant proposals.

Vicente Navarro

Vicente Navarro is unique in this country in health services research and health policy because as a social analyst he uses Marxist rather than Weberian concepts and methods. Therefore, class necessarily becomes a major variable in social change and improvement, but hardly the only one. Navarro is distressed by being regarded as a stereotypical Marxist; many social scientists in this country do not fully understand Marxism as a theory, and those who take off from Weber are not called Weberians (telephone interview, October 3, 1988, and personal correspondence, December 8, 1988; see also Navarro, 1985).

Navarro is professor of health policy at the School of Hygiene and Public Health, Johns Hopkins University, and editor of the *International Journal of Health Services*. One of his major complaints is that he is subjected "to more than my share of offensive and abusive ideologically oriented reviews that, unfortunately, hinder the possibility of establishing a meaningful debate between my position and the positions of other scholars."

I have read Navarro's reviews of the writings of scholars he may not agree with, but he is not abusive. He was mildly critical of one of my own books (Anderson, 1972) because I had paid insufficient attention to class as a variable, but his review was generally favorable and more than I expected from a Marxist-oriented social analyst. Navarro is a prolific writer on health planning in Sweden, on the British National Health Service, and on medical care and capitalism. Favorable reviews of his work come mainly from Europe.

Of course, it is very difficult to carry on a meaningful debate between opposite ideologies, such as democratic capitalism and democratic socialism. The protagonists start from different premises, concepts, and methods of social analysis, which are difficult to fit into one framework. For the purposes of this book, suffice it to make this simplified observation: most social scientists, including myself, are steeped in interest-group liberal democratic thinking; perhaps many of us do not make our position as explicit as Navarro makes his.

Navarro reports having had difficulty getting funding for his research from sources in the United States. He feels that he is judged by standards different from those applied to "mainline" researchers. European funding sources seem to him more "fair"; funding sources in the United States are "ideologically tinged." Hence, his funding sources (such as the German Marshall Fund) are mostly abroad. At the School of Hygiene and Public Health, he observes, high fund raisers get higher salaries.

Nevertheless, Navarro feels that he has a constituency in the United States, among students and others, that sustains him. (I have observed that at meetings of the American Public Health Association he always has a cluster of younger people around him, absorbed in discussion.) He is a health adviser to Jesse Jackson. He is also a member of the Physicians' Committee for National Health Insurance, which was recently organized in Boston. In my health policy classes, I assign material from Navarro, to parallel my usual interest-group, liberal democratic, incremental approach to how policy is formulated in the United States. Navarro claims that, in general, faculty teaching health policy courses ignore his writing. I asked Navarro how he would define himself. He identifies himself with sociology and political sociology.

Summary

What patterns seem to emerge so far in applied research as it is related to social policy? I believe that the researchers discussed here reflect the implicit and explicit values of the general group of social scientists in the United States, as expressed in their choices of problems for research and in their policy preferences.

One overall generalization can be made: all the researchers discussed are, with varying degrees of intensity, social mission–oriented. They want to improve society and its institutions through what one of them called "truth telling." Facts would be the basis of a rational reform of society in the direction of equity, humaneness, and participatory democracy. Researchers like Roemer and Sheps start with an a priori mental model of health services and conduct investigations to promote that model. They regard themselves mainly as advocates, using data honestly and judiciously for their mission.

Most of the researchers would probably start with what already exists: How do institutions work? What are the public's perceptions of illness? What are the characteristics of poverty? What ought to exist must be grounded in the possible, on the basis of learning about how the social system works. A few researchers (Andersen and Shortell, for example) are more likely to conceptualize models for later empirical testing. A few others, such as Greenlick and Fleming, seem to think more in terms of research-administration strategies, since they work in operating agencies.

There is a wide range of research approaches, from essentially descriptive studies ("This is what the animal looks like") to sophisticated statistical studies and model building. The range of disciplines is also wide, and there is interdisciplinary research; this style is regarded as the desirable one in health services research.

Another overall generalization is that all the researchers discussed here except one are basically embedded in the prevailing ideology of liberal democracy and interest-group politics as a means of carrying out social reform, but hardly any make their ideological positions explicit. It does not seem to be necessary: We all breathe the same air, so why examine its composition?

The researchers can be roughly classified from so-called liberal to conservative (tending toward liberal or left-liberal in the American context). They may be impatient with the slow pace of change, but they accept the process. I do not believe that there are any right-wing (that is, extremely market-oriented) conservatives among them. An interesting and very American example of one who operates in the "vital center" is Ginzberg. The exception, of course, is Navarro, who has the temperament and the conviction to espouse the general Marxist position on social systems and power relations—a position that, from the Marxist perspective, would also be reflected in popular elections, if only the population would realize the "false consciousness" underlying its behavior.

The interface between research findings and their use by policymakers and administrators is constantly problematic. Some members of Congress have criticized social researchers for qualifying their results too much. Policymakers and administrators want one-handed researchers, who do not say, "On the one hand . . ." and "On the other hand. . . .' They want disparate numbers, and they want certainty that is beyond the capacity of the social sciences to provide. Likewise with the news media: social scientists have difficulty explaining their findings in the simplistic terms that the media desire.

Access to data from operating agencies is also a problem

because, in the case of private agencies, of business secrets. Moreover, private and public agencies alike fear being evaluated inadequately and unfairly; the researchers cannot really know enough.

A concluding observation, and a central one, is that researchers are not sufficiently aware of the politics of their research endeavors. They fail to include the slippery variable of interest-group politics in social reform, and solutions are not as self-evident as the facts seem to say.

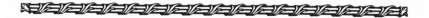

4

The Early Formative Social Environment, 1914-1942

To state a sociological truism, all of us are born at a certain historical time, into a particular family, social segment, and class, and in a certain omnipresent social context. All of us are shaped by a certain training in values and skills, in some gross relation to our personality type, intelligence, and genetic inheritance. All of us must relate to and cope with the available opportunities to satisfy our needs and interests. We live in a moving, relatively unstructured situation, where aspirations can be achieved or not, according to the opportunities. The great majority of us have to adjust and accommodate ourselves to, and essentially accept, the givens of a certain historical period and cope with it (see, for example, Schuman and Scott, 1989). My intention here is to select aspects of my life that are relevant to my career as they relate to the economic, social, and political environment, which was both limiting and liberating, as I perceived it. What I regard as relevant necessarily depends on my decision to err on the side of giving more detail than necessary, rather than too little. Necessary details concern the circumstances that shaped my values and attitudes and how I coped with those circumstances (my bicultural experience, for example). Therefore, I beg the reader's indulgence if at times I personalize my narrative unduly (or, perhaps, do not personalize it enough—for example, with respect to my wife of fifty-one years and my two grown-up children). All the time, I will try to speak of myself as if I were a third person looking at somebody else. (I do, however, think it would be too artificial to refer to myself as *he* rather than *I*. It is for the reader to regard me as someone functioning over a duration of time within a certain period of history.)

The period in which I have lived, 1914–1991, is said to be the most changing, dynamic, and, possibly, psychologically stressful one in human history. Food and shelter have generally been adequate. The driving forces have been applied science and technology and the belief in material progress (and, for some, even in moral progress). For those who were aware and analytical enough about the society with which we have had to cope, there have been choices such as no social system had ever offered before. I presume to believe that I have been one of a generation that became more structurally aware of its surroundings than most have been. I will describe the context and activities of my life from the time I was born to 1942, when I got started in my research career.

I make the sociological and social psychological assumption that there is a relationship (although it may be a very gross and inefficient one) between a person's capacities, education, values, and implanted motivations and the occupational structure at a given time. What has characterized the current century, particularly in the United States, is the great opening of a range of occupational opportunities, an opening facilitated by more education, industrialization, and rural-to-urban mobility. I feel myself very much a part of this process and may even be able to use my life and career as a case example (with no presumption, of course, that generalization from one case is valid). What I have become increasingly conscious of, retrospectively, is my geographical and social mobility into the educational and professional occupational structure. These two kinds of movement have necessitated conscious, almost constant adjustments from rural to urban living styles, from religious orthodoxy to living with cosmic uncertainty (for example, in the over-rationalistic religious denomination of Unitarianism). Culturally, I moved from a densely Norwegian-American enclave in western Wisconsin, where the daily language was a Norwegian dialect, to the culturally pluralistic polyglot called American society (still held together by the English heritage and the New England political and economic philosophies).

I have a powerful sense of my own identity as an individual. I take full responsibility for my actions and behavior, but I still

realize fully that I am also very dependent on a network of supporting relationships. My individualism notwithstanding, as I grew
older I became increasingly humble about how much of my life is
actually under my control. Not much really is, but I have behaved
as if I could shape my life beyond its inherent limitations, by making strategic decisions at what seemed to be convergences of circumstances that I did not shape but could exploit. With this short
prologue I will try to reconstruct the context that shaped my indi-
viduality. As for the nature-nurture interrelationships, I do not presume to be able to unscramble them.

As I said in Chapter One, I believe that my becoming an
orphan at the age of two, with no siblings, generated my propensity
to observe life around me in a semidetached way. My Norwegian
bicultural and bilingual development was another great influence,
as was my very spontaneous interest in wide reading and education,
which began in grade school. All these factors made me, in sociological terms, marginal to my extended family, my age-group peers,
and mainstream American society, with its overwhelmingly English
and New England heritage, as I climbed the educational ladder.

1914–1932

When my parents died, I was already in the care of my father's twenty-two-year-old sister (who later became my foster mother), and I remained on the dairy farm that my paternal grandfather
had founded (see Chapter One). As my consciousness of my extended family and my surroundings expanded, I became aware that
my father's siblings were not my brothers and sisters, and that my
foster mother was not my real mother. My father had left a modest
legacy for me, in the form of life insurance, to be held in trust until
I came of age. Thus, I also became aware that I had my own money.
In due course, I learned that I was in but not of this extended family
and was expected to have a separate destiny from that of my uncles
and aunts. I was not adopted by anyone but was made a ward of the
county, and my legal guardian was the local banker, who managed
my legacy (around $2,000). The banker, according to law, put me
in the custody of my grandmother and my foster mother. My extended family was highly regarded and respected in the community,

and the arrangement for me, almost informal, was that my extended family, under the direction of my grandmother and my foster mother, provided food and shelter and drew on my legacy for clothes and sundries.

Although I cannot remember my parents, I was told a great deal about them, so that they became quite real to me. My father was held up to me as a model of success. He had gone to high school in the village five miles away, walking to and from school in the fall and spring, living on a farm that bordered the village and doing farm chores for room and board in the winter. Very few children, not to mention farm boys, went to high school at that time. This was in 1901. After high school, my father taught in a one-room country school in the area for a couple of years, saved some money, and took off for Minneapolis Business College, a vocational school. From there, he got into the railroad business. He also met my mother in Minneapolis.

I still recall a sea of affectionate support and concern for me. My grandmother and all my uncles and aunts were kind to me. I regarded my foster mother as my mother, although I soon enough found out that she was not. When I was seven years old and had started at the nearby one-room country school, she and her older sister took off for Minneapolis, first to find jobs and then to find spouses. (This was a pattern for women and men alike in the rural areas; the farms could not support the new generation of children. Norwegian immigrants frequently had between six and ten children per family.) The departure of my foster mother was probably more traumatic than I realized at the time, although I do not believe that I suffered any of the psychological damage usually assumed to be associated with that break. Fortunately, my eldest uncle, who was seventeen years my senior and who had been the natural leader of the family enterprise since his father's death, in 1916, spontaneously became my surrogate father. He was then twenty-four years old. We developed an excellent relationship, which persisted throughout his entire life, long after I left the farm. He was a natural leader and a good planner, and he was kind to me. His authority even superseded that of my grandmother, who was, so to speak, the titular head of the household. She had been quite shattered, however, by the loss of her paternalistic husband. She seemed unable to assume her inherited right to run the family. Instead, she deferred to my uncle and surrogate father. He was an excellent model for me. He was clearly his own person, a characteristic I have always admired in others.

Although the farm I grew up on was primarily a dairy farm, with fifteen to twenty milk cows, there were also three draft horses, seventy sheep for wool and mutton for the market, and a hundred or so laying hens for home consumption and the market (a crate of four dozen fresh eggs would be taken to the store in the village, in trade for groceries). This farm, at that time, would have been regarded as a standard middle-range farm, able to sustain a family with adequate food, clothing, shelter, and some amenities. (A thirty-cow farm was considered quite high-class.) This farm was important to my upbringing because the very necessary daily and seasonal routine instilled in the people exposed to it a discipline of unquestioned responsibility. The cows had to be milked twice a day, at the same times each day. The sheep, in the winter, had to be fed daily (in the summer, they were put to pasture). The chickens had to be fed, and the eggs gathered, every day. Seasons came and went, and with them their duties—plowing, planting, harvesting. Until the 1930s, we depended entirely on our wood lots for heating and cooking. Trees had to be cut and sawed and split about a year ahead of time to be ready for the next winter. We learned to accept the eternal verities—to keep cash income flowing and to supply most of our food from the farm itself—and to consider them as in the nature of things. Planning was part of our accommodation to nature; in itself, it was a kind of control through knowledge of what the limits were. To this day, I try to sort out what we have to live with as part of the human condition from what we can do something about.

After my foster mother left, I grew up sharing the farm work wherever I was most needed at the moment, outside or inside the house. There were three grown men on the farm, and so manpower was quite adequate. The womanpower department, however, became overloaded at times because there was only one aunt remaining; she took over the household at the age of sixteen. My grandmother, at fifty, was already suffering from arthritis of the hips. She could not move around or be of much help. This outside-inside experience helped me understand male and female work roles on the farm and gave me an opportunity for participant observation, an experience very few farm boys had at that time.

As long as I carried out my assigned duties and occasional irregular ones, I was left quite to myself. I roamed the meadows and woods with my dog, a collie, while eradicating patches of Canadian thistle, a noxious weed that the cows and sheep would not eat. At the one-room country school, I discovered a small library and exhausted that treasure trove in a short time. After that, I discovered the village Carnegie Library. Every Saturday, I checked out four or more books to read during the week. I hardly did any homework, since I completed all my assignments between class recitations during the day. School was easy, and I stood out from the others by my early and intense academic interest. Fortunately, my teachers—four in seven years (not eight years, because I skipped second grade)— were good teachers and were interested in me. It was almost imprinted on me, from an early age, that I would be going to the village high school and then on to college. My father, as I said, was constantly held up to me as a model, one I had no problem emulating. It never entered my mind to be a farmer or even a skilled worker. Literally all my interests were "intellectual": the humanities, music, but, interestingly, not the "hard" sciences (except to read about their research results for technology).

During several summers in the 1920s, I was exposed to urban life for two to three weeks. My foster mother invited me to visit her and two other aunts, a father's sister and a mother's sister, both living in Minneapolis. I was dazzled by the city, and it got me used to the idea that I was destined to be an urbanite.

I had inherited a large upright piano from my mother; it was shipped to the farm after her death. For three years, beginning when I was eleven, I took piano lessons, first from the local teacher and then from a teacher in high school, during my freshman year. I sang solos and duets in grade school at Christmas parties. I played piano solos at church gatherings—simple numbers, like "To a Wild Rose." My high school piano teacher urged me to go into music and become a pianist. I said I was not good enough: my aspiration was to be a concert pianist or nothing, and I knew I could not attain that level of skill. My teacher persuaded me once to play for the other students at an assembly. I was very nervous. I played a short

Haydn scherzo, but hardly anyone knew who Haydn was (not to mention what a scherzo was). I sang, too, in high school vaudeville performances.

High school was a joy. There were only 115 students in the whole school. My freshman class started in 1928 with 50 students, but only 25 graduated in 1932. I lived in the village as a student boarder during the school week, in three different households over four years. I was really on my own then, but in a small town there is a great deal of informal social control. I felt no constraints, however. I quite accepted the standard mores and never took to smoking or drinking (the latter, at that time, being the main worry of parents). The occasional drunks I saw on the street on Saturday nights in the village were so revolting to me that I stayed away from liquor. Drinking was also illegal. Other students from the surrounding farms, if they were a few miles out, had car pools. In the winter, they lived in town, by some arrangement or other. I bring up this matter of my living in town because this arrangement enabled me to participate in after-school activities (other farm students had to go home for chores), and because I also became part of the village's upper class.

I was comparatively outgoing, and by my second year of high school I was deeply involved in school activities. I was president of the sophomore class. In general, writing was shunned by students, but my own writing ability was sufficiently recognized for me to be the high school reporter for the local weekly and a sports writer (on basketball games) for nearby urban newspapers. The Future Farmers of America (FFA), made up of students (all male) who took the courses in agriculture and intended to be farmers or to do other farm-related work, asked me to be their reporter as well. I recall a glorious field trip with the FFA, in northwest Wisconsin, to look at the big dairy farms in that region.

I continued to be an "intellectual." I got good grades, read omnivorously, and was nurtured by the teachers. Among the other students, I sensed ambivalence about my intellectual interests. These did not seem normal in a boy (not so among the girls, because they could become grade school and high school teachers). The heroes among the boys were the athletes on the basketball team. We had good, competitive basketball teams in those years. In the spring of 1931, we even went to the state tournament, in Madison, but were demolished on the first round—after a season of nineteen straight victories. As for me, I was not varsity material. Although I was physically active, I was no star athlete. To compensate for that deficiency, I became the manager-assistant to the coach for the basketball and field-and-track teams. Thus did I participate for three years in the athletic activities of my high school. I also refereed during practice scrimmages. This is how I blended my intellectual interests with athletics. When I graduated, the local American Legion chapter gave me a medal for being the most outstanding boy in my class of eight boys.

An important incident in my high school education involved an English teacher who took an interest in my apparent language ability. She took me aside one day and said that I spoke good English, but with a Norwegian accent; I should clean it up, in order to get ahead better. Most of the other students also spoke with a Norwegian accent; indeed, even those who could not even speak Norwegian, other than to say *yes* or *no*, had an accent. Knowing my academic aspirations, this teacher wanted to be helpful, and she was. By the time I was at the university, I had consciously cleaned up my speech.

The bicultural, bilingual experience was very important for me because from childhood through high school I was aware of "us" and "them." "We" were Norwegians, and "they" were of Anglo-Saxon origin, as I mentioned in Chapter One. The earliest settlers in the area were from New York State and New England. They constituted the social class who were lawyers, merchants, and politicians, and they established the villages in the area. The European immigrants—in this case, the Norwegians—wanted farmland that the Yankees, as we called them, had already preempted for speculation. The we-they dichotomy was there, but in a rather mild way. Relationships were cordial and constructive, but we Norwegians still had to earn our way into the American Yankee power structure, even though we outnumbered them. By the time I was in high school, I fully realized that I needed to crash this power structure through sheer merit, and cleaning up my accent was a start. Nevertheless, I did not intend or want to repudiate or hide my heritage, for I loved the melodious Norwegian language. To this day, I associate this language with the warmth of family and affection, or with anger and swear words. Even today, in daily family talk, English is not as emotion-laden.

In 1932, I was ready for college. The high school principal helped me with the application papers. He seemed frankly awed that I had ranked in the upper 8 percent of all Wisconsin's graduating classes on a standard knowledge and aptitude test, which had been given for the first time to all students in the state. Only two boys out of the eight in my class went on to college, myself and my best friend, and both of us went to the University of Wisconsin-Madison. My friend quit at the end of his third year. Three of the girls in our class went on to teachers' college.

1932-1942

At the University of Wisconsin, in the fall of 1932, the world opened up for me—intellectually, socially, and politically. The university then had about seven thousand students (the Depression, which began in 1930, had decreased the number of students from ten thousand to seven thousand; by 1938, enrollment was back up to ten thousand). The university was an enormous cornucopia of intellectual outlets, but its enormity could be managed if one found niches congenial to one's interests. My earliest choice of a career was journalism, because of my journalistic activities in high school and the counsel I had sought from teachers. Encouragement had also come from a newspaper reporter who wrote to me and said that he had seen my story on a basketball game in the local press; he thought it was lively.

I enrolled as a student of journalism, in the College of Letters and Science. There were only a few courses directly relevant to journalism. Fortunately, a broad liberal arts education was strongly recommended. The first year, I took a course in reporting. The two local newspapers cooperated with the Department of Journalism to assign students to various events. Students were given access to the pressroom typewriters in the evenings, to meet the next morning's deadlines. It was exciting to pull our fashionable fedoras over our eyes and type up our stories. Sometimes our stories appeared in the papers and sometimes they did not, but this was grass-roots experience. I learned that to climb in the newspaper world, you had to start as a cub reporter before you could become a columnist like Walter Lippmann. I did not feel brash enough to be a cub reporter, because sometimes one had to intrude unduly on the privacy of a would-be informant to get a story, nor did I care to keep unpredictable hours in order to "scoop" an event. My experience in the reporting course was interesting and informative, but I dropped my journalistic aspirations and turned to languages.

During my freshman year, I took Spanish to fulfill the foreign-language requirement for a B.A. degree. I flourished in it. I could roll my r's, thanks to Norwegian, and I could produce firm consonants and vowels. The instructor asked if I had lived in a Spanish-speaking country. I went far enough in Spanish to pass a reading test. I took German concurrently and accumulated enough competence to speak at a daily level and read quite fluently.

Then I moved into Norwegian language and literature, after I learned that there was a professor of Norwegian, Einar Haugen, who had recently arrived on campus. Haugen became a prominent philologist in Norwegian and the other Scandinavian languages. He studied the dialects of Norwegian immigrants in America, as well as the immigrants' adoption of English "loan words" into their native Norwegian (immigrants do this as part of their adjustment to American society and to the physical and technical environment, where they find objects and phenomena for which there are no equivalent words in their native language). I was fascinated enough to compile my own vocabulary of ten thousand words from the dialect spoken on my extended family's farm. About 10 percent of the words were English loan words. Haugen used me as one of many informants from Norwegian immigrant communities in the upper Midwest. I was now in my sophomore year and was casting about for a major. My encounter with Haugen had fired me up and I thought about majoring in Scandinavian-Germanic philology. He cautioned me, however, that there were very few opportunities in academia for philologists, particularly those interested in Norwegian.

I thought next of teaching high school and took an introductory course in education. I dropped the class after a few sessions. It was impossibly dull. Thus, for a while I became an academic "bum," enrolling in courses in economics, philosophy, music appreciation, literature, and whatnot.

I behaved like a member of the leisure class, but without the private income to engage in this luxury indefinitely. I had to stretch the $2,000 that I had brought to the university as far as I could. I was a substitute waiter for several fraternities and sororities. At the end of my sophomore year, in the summer of 1934, I landed an excellent part-time job at the front desk of the university library—a position that eventually led to my career.

I had decided not to go home to the farm for the second summer break of my university sojourn, but to try for a job on campus. I was interviewed by the head of the library's delivery desk, who told me that he could hire me if summer enrollments made this job necessary. While I waited to hear from him, I worked in the Memorial Union cafeteria. I was in charge of distributing dishes and cutlery to the serving areas after items came up the dumbwaiter from the dishwashers in the basement. After I had spent one month on this job, the librarian called me and offered me a job at the delivery desk, fetching books from the stacks for students (stacks were not open at that time). This was a great job, twenty hours a week at thirty-five cents an hour, which I held for four more years, until I earned my M.A. degree. Later, my pay was raised to forty cents an hour. At that time, one could eat quite well for one dollar a day. My room at the YMCA, across the street from the library and next to the Memorial Union, cost me $14.50 a month, with linen and maid service. Thus, I stretched my $2,000 quite comfortably, to cover six years at the university—but back to my academic bumming.

In the second semester of my junior year, in the spring of 1935, I took an advanced introductory course (for juniors up to graduate students) in social psychology. It was given by a well-known professor of sociology, Kimball Young. He was eclectic and a good lecturer. Thus, along with the rest of the class of 250 students, I was exposed to a range of thought, from Freudian psychology to John B. Watson's behaviorism. I was fascinated, in large part because I was learning about myself and my own cultural marginality. With no further reflection, I threw myself into sociology, giving no serious thought to what it might mean in terms of a career. Having learned something about who I was, I then became interested in applied sociology. My major professor, John Gillin, was a well-known criminologist and general expert on social welfare. To accelerate my completing the course requirements for a B.A. in sociology (this new and, at last, permanent interest), I had to attend summer school twice and take an extra semester.

During the 1930s—the days of the Great Depression, as it is now called—the professors and many students were interested in the development of the New Deal, by which President Franklin D. Roosevelt's administration, through massive governmental intervention, was trying to rescue the country. In 1933, when Roosevelt took office, we were at the bottom of the Depression, and there were signs that people might make a run on the banks to withdraw their deposits. Roosevelt quashed that possibility by declaring an indefinite closing of the banks. One could withdraw only enough for daily needs. All my money was in my hometown bank. I thought I was going to be entirely strapped for money, until I learned that I could draw enough for subsistence, as I had always done. Anyway, the atmosphere was glum and fearfully uncertain. Professors and students in the social sciences were taking an interest in problems of economic social policy. Professor Edwin Witte, a labor economist in the university's Department of Economics, was appointed by President Roosevelt to be secretary of the Committee for Economic Security, which formulated what became the Social Security Act of 1935, establishing old-age pensions, unemployment insurance, and related programs. In 1937, back at the university, Witte gave what was probably the first course in social insurance to be taught anywhere, drawing on his work and experience with the Social Security Act. The large enrollment—300 students, myself included—was proof of the great interest in economic social policy among students. (In due course, I earned my M.A. in sociology, in 1938, concentrating on social welfare policy and programs.)

At the University of Wisconsin, I was also involved in extracurricular activities. I was active in the International Club as a representative of the University YMCA. I was president of the Norse Club, a member of the Men's Glee Club, and a member of the Student Progressive Club, a student offshoot of the Progressive Party, founded by Robert M. La Follette, Sr. (his two sons, Philip and Robert, Jr., were the governor of the state and a U.S. senator, respectively). The Student Progressive Club was the largest and most active of the student political clubs of its time. I may have been a marginal person in some respects, but on campus I was not politically marginal; I was politically in the vital center. The Young Communist League (YCL) was quite visible but small, as were the socialist groups. These very left-wing political organizations never seemed to make much headway on campus, but, thanks to the university's liberal tradition of free speech, they were left alone and met in university facilities.

By the spring of 1937, I had my B.A. and my job in the university library, but I had exhausted my legacy. As circumstances would have it, I had two excellent contacts in Oslo, Norway, people I had met at the University of Wisconsin. The first, whom I met in 1935, was Arvid Brodersen, a Rockefeller Foundation fellow in sociology, ten years my senior. The second, whom I met in 1936, had been a graduate student in chemistry at the university. They encouraged me to visit them in Norway.

Although I was broke, I threw all caution to the winds and borrowed $300 from a friend. I took off for eight weeks in Europe, Scandinavia, and the United Kingdom, traveling by bus to New York and by boat to Europe. This was an impressionable trip for a twenty-three-year-old. It set my sights on the possibility of doing social research in Norway. It was also the first of many trips to Europe. I was back in time for the fall term at school, where I was to pursue an M.A. in sociology.

My last year at the university was rough financially, but before leaving for Europe I had been assured of a continuing job in the library. I was also promised a part-time janitorial job in the YMCA, sweeping out the entire ground floor every morning at five o'clock for two weeks each month, which gave me my room. I borrowed $50 from the student-loan fund for my tuition and joined a student-run meal cooperative ($3.75 a week for lunch and dinner each day, dinner only on Sundays). There I also met my wife, Helen, who was as financially strapped as I was. We both graduated in the spring of 1938 and were married a year later. In the meantime, however, much happened that was extremely significant for my future career.

During my last year, I was wondering what I could do with an M.A. in sociology. It was not a professional degree, and the job market for anything at all was extremely bad. The head of the library, Gilbert Doan, must have been watching me, for he asked me to come to his office. He wanted to know what I was going to do after the spring of 1938, and I said I had no idea. My major professor was unable to find anything for me, and I had no intention of doing further graduate work. I had no money and no relatives to fall back on. I was an orphan, completely on my own. Doan suggested that I go to library school and become a college librarian: I already had four years of experience, and the field, which was predominantly female, needed male administrators (a remark that would sound strange today). He said I could go to the University of Michigan's library school, which offered a one-year program in library science to those who already had a B.A. or a B.S. If I could not afford to do that, I could get a full-time job in the library while I was a student and take two years to complete the B.A. in library science. Doan was a graduate of the school and had been on the senior staff there. He said he would be glad to recommend me. I liked academia and books, and I visualized myself as a college librarian, working in a congenial environment.

In June 1938 I hitchhiked to Ann Arbor, where I was interviewed by the associate librarian, a pleasant man who said that he could not promise me a job right then but that I should come back in the fall. If there was a job then, it would pay $86 a month, and the thirty-seven hours a week would be planned around my courses. I hitchhiked back to Madison and worked at the library there during the summer.

What to do if I could not get the library job at the University of Michigan? I borrowed $400 from my surrogate father on the farm and prepared to go to Ann Arbor and enroll in the library school, without a job. When I arrived, however, I was told that I had a job.

My first year in library school and in my job went by quickly and quite pleasantly. I missed sociology, and so I got acquainted with a few graduate students in the department, one of whom became my lifelong friend. My fiancée and I wanted to get married, but I could not support her. After some effort, she got a part-time skilled-typing job in the catalogue department of the law library.

In my second year, we married and set up housekeeping in a small apartment near the campus, living very prudently on $125 a month.

I earned my B.A. in the spring of 1940 but could not find a library job. I kept the job I had and enrolled in the University of Michigan's graduate school, for a Ph.D. in sociology. (I had learned that the college librarian without a faculty appointment could talk more easily with professors if he or she had a Ph.D.) I was in graduate school part-time; fortunately, the library's personnel policy seemed to be that I could have my modest job as long as I was a student.

During the 1941–42 academic year, I went through an awful crisis for someone working in the "whispering profession," as librarianship has sometimes been called. An infection in my left middle ear required a massive mastoidectomy, which meant the total loss of hearing in that ear. I might have been fired, but the library administration limited my front-desk duties and increased my work behind the scenes (for example, supervising the collating of newspapers for binding).

This chapter shows that I was an aggressive, risk-taking person who coped with marginality. I depended completely on myself for survival. My career, too, has reflected my marginality within a constantly changing occupational structure that continually has opened up opportunities with uncertain futures.

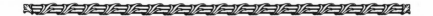

5

Beginning
a Fifty-Year Career,
1942–1952

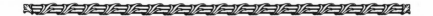

Early in 1942, several months after I had recovered from my mastoidectomy, there was a call to the library school from Nathan Sinai, a professor of public health, asking if we had anyone with a background in both social science and library skills. When I met with Sinai, he showed me many boxes of books and articles he had been collecting for fifteen years, in the hope of establishing a unit in medical care and a health services research library. Sinai saw a relatively diminishing role for traditional public health if the field did not recognize the emerging problem of chronic illness and the possibility of fusing preventive and curative medicine. Now he had received a developmental grant of $7,000 from the Kellogg Foundation. His first need was to get his books and articles organized in a library format—catalogued and classified for ready access. Within a week, I was working as a research assistant in the first unit at any university anywhere in the country to be conducting research on health services delivery and related problems. My salary was increased, from $86 a month to $125, or $1,500 a year.

By July, I had established the library, complete with card catalogue and arrangements of shelved books and files of clippings that we called "fugitive facts," organized by subject matter. I had a part-time secretary to do the typing. Everything had to be done absolutely from scratch—the arranging of catalogue cards, shelves, and files, the subscribing to a dozen or so journals that followed trends in the health field. We ordered relevant books as they were published. An added bonus for me was that, while classifying the books and articles on medical care that Sinai had assembled over the years, I became acquainted with virtually all the literature on medical care in six months.

As I was approaching the end of my task, Sinai joked that I had worked myself out of a job. What was I going to do next? I told him that an idea for a research project had come to me while I was establishing the library. In my review of the literature, I had seen that the rapidly emerging nonprofit Blue Cross and Blue Shield plans were having problems because they were considered to be insurance companies and were therefore subject to the same regulations that governed stock companies. Those regulations mandated rather high financial reserves, to back up insurance contracts and ensure solvency. The hospital-sponsored Blue Cross plans and the medical society–sponsored Blue Shield plans had no such capital, however. There was already enough public and legislative interest in the Blue nonprofit plans that state after state was enacting special enabling legislation, as it was called, to exempt the Blue plans from maintaining large cash reserves and paying corporate taxes. The emergence of this special legislation had never been analyzed, and I proposed to study its emergence and rationale within the regulatory laws on insurance.

The Blue plans avoided the word *insurance;* they used *prepayment* instead. (Operationally, of course, they were insurance, but law can reify reality.) I spent months in the law library, poring over the statutes of the approximately forty states that had passed enabling legislation. In due course, this research was published (Anderson, 1944) as the first report in a series that Sinai established for what became known in 1944 as the Bureau of Public Health Economics within the School of Public Health. (The bureau's only professional personnel were a doctor of public health and a sociologist; we did not think of asking the Department of Economics for permission to use the word *economics* in the bureau's name.) This publication was in relatively great demand, considering its narrowness; it is still being quoted far and wide.

Early in 1943, after I had worked with Sinai for a year, I suffered another crisis in my already deficient hearing. My right ear developed a severe mastoid infection, apparently stemming from infections I had had as a child. I underwent another massive mastoidectomy, performed by the same surgeon who had operated on my left ear. This operation left me with stable but deficient hearing, which of course would make teaching difficult. Sinai was very sympathetic. He said that I certainly could do research and maintain the library. As fate would have it, however, the electronics industry, stimulated by World War II, began to apply elements of radio communications technology to the design of hearing aids. At almost the precise time when I needed a hearing aid, good ones were on the market. Shortly after I had recovered fully from the second operation, I bought a hearing aid. For all practical purposes, it restored my hearing; my auditory nerves were normal, and all I needed was amplification along the entire hearing spectrum.

I assisted Sinai in organizing a couple of new courses in health services administration. I produced conceptual and factual syllabi, a task I could carry out quite easily because of my growing knowledge of the field. After a while, Sinai actually went on leave and delegated a course to me for one semester.

It was a challenging experience to establish a new academic field, and Sinai was exciting to work with. He was in the thick of the activities surrounding the voluntary health insurance plans that were emerging and the federal health insurance bills that were proposed in every term of Congress. (He had first become interested in medical care when he was a technical staff member of CCMC; see page xv). In 1944, the same year that the Bureau of Public Health Economics was established, Sinai was a consultant to Washington State's welfare department. The state had a medical program for the recipients of old-age assistance, a means-tested pension program plus medical care. This program was innovative in that the department of welfare contracted with the medical bureaus of the county medical societies for physicians' services. The bureaus had arisen in response to the practice of contract medicine in the area, whereby groups of physicians sold contracts to industry—a procedure that was anathema to mainstream medicine. Later on, the bureaus were a response to government-funded health insurance. The innovation was in the government's contracting with a physician-sponsored medical plan for recipients of old-age assistance, who were covered along with other plan members (the latter were groups of employees, as in private insurance plans). The elderly people had free

choice of physician, just as the others did. It was particularly interesting to Sinai that here was a large group of older people whose
use of services could be studied. He was looking ahead to the time
when the elderly would become an increasingly large proportion of
the population, and to the implications for chronic illness and
long-term care, including institutional care. Washington's program
presented a natural laboratory.

When Sinai returned from his consultancy in Washington,
he asked if I would be interested in spending the summer of 1945
in that state, to make a thorough study of how the plan for the
elderly was working. This would be a research and policy contribution to the health field. I jumped at the chance. I thought I could
get a summer research grant from the graduate school for travel and
incidental expenses, and so I wrote up my first grant application,
stating my objectives and explaining my project's relevance to the
health field. The grant was awarded.

I took my wife and one-and-a-half-year-old daughter with me
to Olympia, Washington, and was assigned to the director of the
program, a physician. I was given office space and access to all the
records. Out of twenty-one counties, I selected seven for intensive
investigation. I also visited the administrators of the medical bureaus and selected physicians for background information.

This study became my first major fieldwork. When I had
finished it, I presented an overview of data and impressions to the
administrative staff of the welfare department. It was published in
our research series and was in great demand (Anderson, 1947). For
the first time, there were fairly detailed data on use and expenditures
for this segment of the population. The eligibility requirements for
old-age assistance were so liberal that the majority of the state's
elderly were in the program, and so it was quite representative of
the entire group. I did a follow-up study on physicians' involvement in the program as well (Anderson, 1948).

In the mid 1940s, Sinai was also a consultant to the governor
of California, Earl Warren (later chief justice of the U.S. Supreme
Court). Sinai not only helped the governor draft a universal health
insurance bill for California but also testified on behalf of the governor and the bill before a state legislative committee. This was a
traumatic experience for Sinai, however; the committee attempted

to discredit his expertise because one of his degrees happened to be in veterinary medicine. "So, you are a horse doctor?" one of the committee members laughed. The bill did not even get to the floor of the legislature. Sinai was quite shaken. His experience taught me that if I wished to engage in health services research, a lot of which was inherently controversial, I ought not engage in consulting politicians. Rather, I should maintain a low political profile and produce data for relevant policy purposes. I could consult behind the scenes, as a sort of gray eminence, but I would not testify for or against a particular bill. In the case of what happened to Sinai, someone else—a sympathetic member of the legislature, for example—should have testified on behalf of the governor. I am sure that Sinai's research ambitions for health services were damaged thereafter, although he did expand his staff, who produced useful studies. He had already had his difficulties with medical associations and politically active physicians, because of his apparent sympathy with the idea of government health insurance in some form. Sinai was also sympathetic to the movement for voluntary health insurance and was willing to see if it would work. (He was an essentially pragmatic person; during this time, and far into the 1960s, one was supposed to be against government intervention in health services, and for the voluntary approach as a compromise.) Many physicians were against health insurance of any kind, although some prominent medical leaders did support voluntary insurance.

Shortly after the Bureau of Public Health Economics was established, Sinai and the dean of the School of Public Health sponsored three conferences at the school. The first was on current problems and issues in voluntary health insurance and the current status of federal legislation for government health insurance. The second was for faculty in preventive medicine at medical and public health schools. The third was on dental public health. Each of the three was the first national conference on its particular problem.

The conference on health insurance was the controversial and lively one, because of the apparent imminence, evident in bills proposed in Congress, of some form of government health insurance. There were representatives from the private insurance companies, the Blue Cross–Blue Shield plans, and the group-practice prepayment plans, as well as proponents of government health insurance. The nonprofit Blue plans resented the intrusion of the for-profit insurance companies; until the mid 1940s, the Blue plans had the market to themselves, state by state. Leaders from the Blue plans scolded the for-profit plans for making money on sickness. The group-practice prepayment plans criticized mainstream health insurance and the fee-for-service system for being inefficient and costly and said that health services should be organized into group-practice prepayment units. The proponents of government health insurance proclaimed that only a universal, government-sponsored health insurance plan would solve the problems of cost and equal access to all, regardless of income and residence. For a novice like me, this conference was a great experience in learning what the real political and medical issues were. I also got to meet the elite among the leaders of the health and health insurance fields.

The conference on preventive medicine was also of great interest and significance, for it brought together in one meeting the leading (and struggling) faculties of preventive medicine, which was a stepchild of clinical medicine. There has been an increase in its status since then, but the clinical specialties still have higher status. There were debates on how preventive medicine should be taught in medical schools—as a specialty, or as an attitude and philosophy in the daily handling of patients. Again, as also in the third conference, I met the elite.

The third conference was less lively because public health dentists and privately practicing dentists were able to reach consensus more easily on appropriate strategies for maintaining the dental health of the public. I believe that my exposure to these conferences kindled in me the concept of being practice-oriented as well as academically oriented. I learned the respective cultures. Ever since, I have felt able to interact with them as an accepted outsider.

As he showed by his work for Washington State, Sinai was an opportunist, always on the lookout for "natural laboratories." He grasped another such opportunity through the Emergency Maternity and Infant Care (EMIC) program.

As World War II progressed and the United States entered the conflict, men were inducted into the military services. Recall that there was no universal health insurance in the United States. Private health insurance was covering only a minority of the people, and maternity care was usually excluded—because it was regarded as predictable. Congress, in its wisdom, passed the EMIC act, to help the wives and small children of men in the armed services. They were provided with free maternity and infant services, both preventive and curative. This program became, in effect, the first national health services program. It was administered by the Department of Labor's Children's Bureau through the state health departments. A reimbursement method had to be devised to pay obstetricians, pediatricians, generalists, and hospitals, and quality standards had to be formulated.

Sinai raised enough grant money to mount a research project for studying the administration of the EMIC program. The objective of the study was to analyze the administrative problems encountered in mounting a national health services program through state departments of health. What were the practical methods of reimbursing hospitals and physicians? How were standards of quality formulated and applied? The results of the study became a reference point for developing methods—including government funding—to reimburse hospitals and physicians. A staff of four, including me, was assembled. We spent several weeks in the Children's Bureau. The rest of the staff fanned out in selected states, but I was kept in Ann Arbor. (I was apparently being held in reserve for the Washington State study that I have already described. It was a more than satisfactory trade-off for me in that I got my own project.) Later, I was Sinai's coauthor for the EMIC report (Sinai and Anderson, 1948). A key staff member who was to write the bulk of the report left for another job. I was thus given the major responsibility for writing up the study. (Sinai suggested that I be the senior author, but I said that was ridiculous. His offer was typical of his generosity toward his staff, and I have tried to emulate him with my research staffs ever since.)

While all this activity was going on, I was going through a rocky time. In 1945, I failed four of five preliminary Ph.D. exams. In itself, failing was hardly unusual in the sociology department, and I was given another chance at the four examinations. I myself did not feel that I had done well. I realized that I was too far outside the department and not sufficiently integrated as a graduate student; I was not completely tuned in to the department's culture. My problem was structural, not personal. I did not have any strong tie with a professor in the department. There was also some question about the relevance of public health (the area in which I was working) to sociology. I took the examinations again in 1946, and this time I failed two of the four. The department seemed confused about how to handle my case. I was called in for a hearing before the whole department and got permission to try again, but the faculty's reservations were palpable (except on the part of one very senior professor, who urged me not to quit). I consulted with Sinai, who I felt was my real mentor, and said I could not take any more; I was going to quit and seek employment outside academia, in health programs (I had become quite familiar with operational problems). Sinai shot back with unequivocal personal advice (not his usual style), which I never forgot and have applied ever since. He said, "The Department of Sociology is so confused about you that the faculty did not stop you arbitrarily, but would rather that *you* make the decision to quit. In such a situation, you should continue to force the faculty to make such a decision, and not you. Go back for the last try, because if you do not, you will live all the rest of your life with irresolution." I went back for the final trial. A few days after the examinations, the head of the department called me and reported that I had passed and even done well.

The next hurdle was my dissertation. I proposed to do a study on the emergence of health insurance in the United States as a social movement. My several years with Sinai had given me an opportunity to get to know the literature on this topic, and it would also represent original research in that no one had done this before. I was asked to suggest a committee, and I did. It included a professor of economics who specialized in social insurance; Sinai, as a specialist in medical care and public health; and three sociologists. My proposal was accepted, and the chairman, who regarded himself as a "situation analyst," told me that he would be my devil's advocate. The dissertation process went very smoothly. I turned in nine chapters for comments, three chapters at a time. Surprisingly, I did not get any comments. My dissertation was accepted and commended. The dissertation hearing late on that afternoon in February 1948 was very congenial, in contrast to what it had been during the series of examinations. This is why I conclude that my problem was structural, rather than personal. I was a marginal type who still had not found a niche in sociology; medical sociology had not been invented.

While working with Sinai, I read, with great interest, three seminal books, which formed a launching pad for my continuing formulation of research projects in the health field and my subsequent synthetical writing. They were *The Development of Modern Medicine: An Interpretation of the Social and Scientific Factors Involved,* by Richard H. Shryock ([1936] 1979); *The Incidence of Illness and the Receipt and Costs of Medical Care Among Representative Families: Experiences in Twelve Consecutive Months During 1928–1931,* by I. S. Falk, Margaret C. Klem, and Nathan Sinai (1933); and *Health and Environment,* by Egar Sydenstricker (1933). The first book introduced me to the panorama of the history of medicine in its social context. The second book brought me into the mainstream with respect to data on family expenditures for health services, use of services, and morbidity patterns. The third book exposed me to concepts of disease and its related social factors. These books, added to my macrosociological orientation, laid the groundwork for my research.

The Bureau of Public Health Economics subscribed to many journals, which I was supposed to peruse for relevant articles and trends. As an almost incidental spinoff of this activity, I started composing a monthly abstract, and I had the first two issues ready by the time the conference on preventive medicine was held. Some participants saw those abstracts and suggested that they should have general circulation. The result was a periodic abstract of articles and events, which interested parties subscribed to. It was called *Public Health Economics.* (Long after my departure from the bureau, this project became *Medical Care Review,* with the addition of original articles. It is now published by the Health Administration Press but is still based in the School of Public Health in Ann Arbor. I have found this publication a tremendously timesaving resource.)

After 1945, the School of Public Health was training many physicians for public health and teaching posts who had returned from military duty. One of them was C. Edward Hobbs, a psychiatrist from London, Ontario, who had been sent to Ann Arbor by the Faculty of Medicine at the University of Western Ontario to study for a master of public health (M.P.H.) degree. He was then to return to the University of Western Ontario and take over the new Department of Clinical Preventive Medicine, where he would expose medical students to the social aspects of medicine. Hobbs and I got to know each other well. He was eight years my senior and was in the courses that Sinai and I cotaught. He would drop into my office to chat about medical care, public health, health insurance, and related topics. There turned out to be a specific reason for his chats: he was looking for a sociologist to join his department in the medical school at the University of Western Ontario. He said that I was the only sociologist he knew who made any sense; I believe that I was the only sociologist he had ever known.

In 1947, after Hobbs got his M.P.H., he went back to Ontario and started his new job. One day, I got a telephone call from him. He wondered if I would consider joining the medical faculty in his department. I said I would like to consider the offer, and I went to Ontario, where I found the opportunity and the setting quite appealing. We had more telephone conversations, and I made another visit. This process took over a year. The job description expanded, shaped by whatever experience, knowledge, and interests I could bring to this new endeavor. Finally, I accepted the offer—but not before discussing it with Sinai and my wife.

Sinai simply said, "Glad to have known you." (This response contrasted with what he had said when Washington State's welfare department made me a tentative offer, after I had worked on the project there. On that occasion, he said, "After a year there, you will have nothing left but the scenery.")

My wife and I now had two children. Helen, being a loyal helpmate, was willing to go, even though she was not enthusiastic about moving to a country where they toasted the queen of England. Helen was of New England ancestry on her mother's side. Her forebears had helped to settle New England and supported the American Revolution. There had been a whole colony in New England, known as the United Empire Loyalists, who fled to Ontario and opposed the American Revolution; but if the move furthered my career, she would go, too.

I was turning down a promotion to assistant professor, but I gambled that being on the faculty of a medical school would enhance my career. The pay increase was not particularly substantial, although we were helped by the lower cost of living in Canada. Before I left Ann Arbor, I had been earning around $4,000, plus fringes, and Helen was a full-time homemaker. In the Canadian post, I earned $5,000 a year, plus fringes. I gather that this salary was average for sociologists in 1949. One had to be very prudent—no car, for example.

With Hobbs's assistance and participation, I was to organize a course for first-year medical students. A few extra lectures on health insurance and medical care organization were also to be given. With the modest research funds available, I was to start some relevant research in social medicine. I would be an associate professor, in charge of teaching the social aspects of medicine within the Department of Clinical Preventive Medicine. I was to start on January 1, 1949. Helen and I had another child due late in January, however, and so I was permitted to wait until after his birth, which occurred on February 10, 1949. (I could not have taken my family to Ontario yet in any case, because first I had to find a house to rent.) I went over to London shortly after our son's birth and rented a room near the medical school. I still had to find a house, which turned out to be difficult, and to organize a course for the fall semester. Hobbs asked how much time I wanted before I started teaching, and I said six months, which was granted.

During those six months, I started to read the literature on epidemiology in the medical library. (At Michigan, I had covered the literature on medical care delivery systems.) The course content for the first-year students was to include mortality and morbidity patterns over time and geographical regions, as well as social correlates for many specific diseases. Hobbs thought that the medical students should be exposed to the overall background of mortality and morbidity before entering the clinical years; medical students to this day are notoriously indifferent to epidemiology because it deals with groups of people, rather than with individuals. Hobbs's strategy was to lead off with the clinical characteristics of a particular prevalent disease, such as diabetes. I would follow with its morbidity and mortality characteristics. I organized a rather elaborate syllabus on patterns of mortality and morbidity for communicable diseases and on maternal and infant mortality. As I recall, one student asked me what value all this information would have for his future practice. I told him that it could be used for prognosis. That answer seemed to satisfy the first-year students, for the question was not raised again.

I regard myself mainly as a sociologist in the structural-functionalist mode, a style that lends itself to analysis of systems (such as health services), mortality and disease patterns in populations over time and space, and associated stages of social development and cultures. I thought, as Hobbs did, that, as a strategic beginning, it was the better part of wisdom in a department of preventive medicine not to introduce social science overtly—and the students were hardly aware that I was introducing social science. I could have participated in clinical rounds and observed physicians' and patients' behavior. At this early stage, however, I did not want to intrude on clinical matters, although it would have been interesting. Strategically, I thought it was too soon for the first full-time academic sociologist in a medical school to do that. I quite studiously avoided behaving like a physician. For example, I never wore a white laboratory coat (although, if I had gone on clinical rounds, I would have done so, to camouflage my role before the patient). I intended to be my own unambiguous person and enact my own role. If I had stayed longer in this position, I might have investigated role behaviors of physicians and patients, but I would have preferred to engage an ethnographer (or what sociologists call a symbolic interactionist) for that purpose. Analytically, as a sociologist, I feel uncomfortable with single cases. Still, I am hardly a sophisticated quantitative sociologist, either. I believe I brought to the school of public health and to the medical school a perspective on what I eventually called the three interrelated problem areas peculiar to medical sociology: population and disease, people and their attitudes toward health and health professionals, and the institutional structure that was developed to cope with the two foregoing problems. All three of these areas are heavily sociological in emphasis. I believe that I also became an amateur economist and political scientist in investigating need, demand, and the service structure, perhaps adequately enough for the level of abstraction I was working with to open up a new field of research. In time, I expected, younger scholars would come along, with sharper concepts and tools of investigation than I would ever possess; and this has happened.

I believe that Hobbs and I were a successful team. He was my sponsor and legitimated me for the students (and faculty). The president of the university, a physician and former dean of the medical school, also strongly supported my role.

During the six months when I was not teaching, I visited selected people in medicine and public health in Toronto and Montreal. The previous year, on my way back from Seattle, Washington, I had returned to Ann Arbor by way of Vancouver, Regina, and Winnipeg, where I had former colleagues, whom I told about my plans to move to Ontario and work with Hobbs. My reception was warm, east and west: Hobbs was known and respected all over Canada.

My position on the medical faculty was financed by a five-year grant from the Morrow Foundation, in Toronto. (During part of this grant period, and at the end of it, my position was to be absorbed into the general funding of the medical school and the university. In addition, if I were interested in taking over the position of the only sociologist in the university, who was in the Department of Economics and Political Science, I was welcome to do so; he was approaching retirement. As a starter in that department, I gave a course in social and health insurance.) As part of my career pattern, it should be noted, I continued to be financed by philanthropic foundation grants; universities were not ready to draw from their general funds to finance my kind of interest and the competence wanted by academic entrepreneurs like Sinai and Hobbs.

My light teaching load enabled me to spend a great deal of time on my research interests, as was intended. In collaborating with Hobbs, I had access to a fund of $20,000 for research, more than before. My research into preexisting, unexplored historical data on population, mortality, and disease resulted in articles in good journals. I showed that mortality rates for age groups above infancy had been falling in the latter nineteenth century, before the advent of public health and personal health services. My explanation for this fall in mortality rates was a stabilized food supply due to better transportation, among other factors (Anderson, 1953a, 1955). I also helped to open up long-term historical trends in infant mortality, demonstrating that a shift had taken place from environmental to biogenetic causes of infant mortality as rates fell rapidly in the early twentieth century (Anderson, 1953b). As something of a sideline, I wrote an article (Anderson, 1952) describing my strategy and tactics in introducing sociology into a medical school. It has been cited quite often.

With the research fund that I have mentioned, I was able to hire a statistician to study morbidity patterns in a group of subscribers to a comprehensive medical plan in Windsor, Essex County, Ontario, across the river from Detroit. Nathan Sinai, as early as in the late 1930s, had been a consultant to the Essex County Medical Society, which organized one of the first comprehensive health insurance plans for recipients of public assistance. The Province of Ontario entered into a contract with Windsor Medical Services, as it was called, an innovation in that a public agency was contracting with a private agency to carry out a public responsibility. Eventually, Windsor Medical Services offered membership to anyone in Essex County. This research, a pioneer effort to learn something about which illnesses prompted people to seek physicians' services, was a study of demand within a plan that did not charge patients anything at the time of service (Smiley, Buck, Anderson, and Hobbs, 1954).

After a couple of years, I felt quite integrated into the University of Western Ontario, with my base in the medical school and outreach to other relevant units of the university. Still, it seemed unlikely that I would stay there indefinitely. Much as my wife and I enjoyed London, Ontario, as a family town, she wanted to return to the United States eventually, and I intuitively felt that perhaps the base (that is, the critical mass) was not large enough for my type of research interest. If there were opportunities in universities in the United States, I would probably return.

For several years after the end of World War II, the World Health Organization (WHO) set up a number of fellowships for physicians from the United States who were associated with preventive medicine (or social medicine, as it became the style to call it), so that they could spend a summer in northern Europe, Great Britain, and Scandinavia, visiting professors in medical schools and in departments of public health who were working in social medicine.

WHO wished to open up an interchange between Europe and the United States after the long break during the war. I decided to apply for one of these fellowships, even though I felt I would be passed over because I was not a physician. Apparently on the strength of my being in a department of preventive medicine and doing the kind of research I was doing, I was accepted. By this time, I had become somewhat well known in the "social medicine" field. In the summer of 1951, I sent my family to a lakeside cottage near Milwaukee, to stay with relatives, and I spent three glorious and informative months in Great Britain, Denmark, Norway, and Sweden. WHO made all the arrangements in each country, which in turn made appointments with relevant people. While I was in Europe, I met Cecil G. Sheps. He was also a WHO fellow, and we were paired in Great Britain and Sweden for the same appointments. We got to know each other well. Being a WHO fellow meant easy access and helpful conversations on what was going on in these countries. The WHO fellowship inspired me to move into cross-national research in health services delivery systems, if I could find the money for it.

When I returned in the fall, I entered my third year at the University of Western Ontario. Early in 1952, Cecil Sheps wrote to me from the University of North Carolina School of Public Health and Medical School and asked if I would be interested in a position as medical sociologist in the medical complex. I said I was interested, and I was flown down to Chapel Hill in February 1952. I spent three days in intensive interviews with twenty-two people in public health, medicine, and sociology. From the standpoint of the development of medical sociology at this time, the position was an important one. By this time, I had been on the faculties of a school of public health and a school of medicine, and I had a Ph.D. in sociology. Sheps was enthusiastic about the possibility of my coming to the University of North Carolina. He (as a physician in social medicine) and I (as a sociologist with my experience) thought alike. I felt very favorably received by everyone, particularly by the academics in the medical complex. I went back to Ontario to wait for what seemed to be a sure offer. For several weeks, nothing was happening, and I had to make a decision about Hobbs and my future with him.

Finally, Sheps wrote and called to report an unexpected difference of opinion about me between the medical people and the sociology department. The impression I got, difficult to verify, was that the medical people thought I had a good grasp of health and medical problems (although I was a sociologist), but the sociologists wanted someone more theoretically oriented than I was. There was probably also the question of a foundation subsidy, which was not feasible in my case.

Again, as at the University of Michigan, I saw my problem as structural, rather than personal. I was not a "real" sociologist, although I was regarded as productive in health services research. The medical people, I am sure, felt that I knew their problems; perhaps the sociologists felt that I was somewhat co-opted. This was a sobering experience for me. I believed that I had chosen the correct seminal experiences to be a medical sociologist, but I had never had a "pure" sociology identity in a field that is exceedingly conscious of creating a disciplinary identity. Academically, I was in limbo. What kind of career line could I follow?

Not long after that, I had a long and persuasive letter from Kenneth Williamson, executive secretary of the Health Information Foundation, in New York City, about a position as research director. I had heard about the foundation, which was chartered in 1950 as a nonprofit educational agency by the drug, pharmaceutical, and chemical industries. Its purpose was to finance and promote research on the health services of the United States. Williamson knew of me and my background and felt that I had the qualifications the foundation wanted. If I were interested, the foundation would bring me to New York for an interview.

Being a New Deal liberal, nurtured during the long Roosevelt administration, I was suspicious of big business. As for the drug, pharmaceutical, and chemical industries, I assumed that they would have a self-serving interest in promoting research primarily intended to extol the American health services and ward off some form of government health insurance, which I knew those industries opposed, as did the American Medical Association. I was quite committed to universal health insurance, but, like Nathan Sinai, I was pragmatic enough to support voluntary health insurance and see how far it could go to cover the population. For several reasons—to be fair, not to prejudge the motives for the establishment of the Health Information Foundation, to indulge my natural curiosity, and not to turn down any opportunity in advance—I accepted the invitation to go to New York. I went there with a chip on my shoulder. I intended to be very aggressive in finding out what kind of research context I would be working in with respect to objectivity, freedom to select research topics, and freedom to publish whatever the results might be.

When I arrived at the foundation's headquarters, Williamson took me in hand. He gave me a very straightforward description of the foundation's objectives and financing and of the public service philosophy of the industry and the foundation's board of directors. The board was made up of the presidents of the major drug, pharmaceutical, and chemical firms in the United States. (I had feared that the board members would be public relations directors, beholden to their employers.) The foundation had been more or less foundering on the question of how it could mount a program of research and information that would get national attention from politicians, health policymakers, professional health associations, the voluntary health insurance industry, and academic researchers in social science. The foundation had an annual budget of around $500,000 for research and media information on the American health services. So far, however, a viable research program had not been developed. Williamson had been a worker in the health field, mostly in association work, for a number of years before the foundation was established, and he had been an assistant to the executive director of the American Hospital Association. He hoped that voluntary health insurance could be the backbone of health insurance for the American people, with government subsidies for the poor administered by private agencies, such as Blue Cross and Blue Shield.

At that time, the only source of basic information on the health services was the Bureau of Research and Statistics, in what was then the Social Security Administration. The bureau was headed by I. S. Falk, who had been on the technical staff of CCMC and was a coauthor of the household survey, with Sinai and Margaret Klem. Falk, as a U.S. civil servant, was a well-known and ardent proponent of government health insurance and testified in favor of it before committees of Congress. The business and professional health associations were suspicious of the extensive data produced by Falk's bureau on the costs and operations of voluntary health insurance. His data stood the test of scrutiny, but no matter—its source was still suspect. Falk's implicit interpretation of the data was that the glass was half empty, rather than half full; in fact, he said it was over two-thirds empty. The industry supporting the foundation felt that there should be more than a single source of data and research for controversial policy issues. Hence, the foundation was created.

I was also interviewed by the president of the foundation, W.H.P. Blandy. He had been admiral of the American Atlantic fleet during World War II. After the war, he was admiral of the fleet that was guarding the atomic tests in the Bikini Atoll, in the South Pacific. He had learned how to work with physical scientists. Despite the exemplary behavior of the American military under civilian control during World War II, I was somewhat fearful of formulating a research program that would draw mainly on the social sciences and report to a military person, but it did not take me long to be disabused of this stereotype, at least in Blandy's case. I asked Blandy right away what he expected of a research director, and the answer came right back: "To formulate and conduct a research program to assist in the understanding and improvement of the American health services." The interview is still vivid in my memory. I was to originate research ideas and projects on the basis of the broad aims of the foundation, and they certainly were broad. I asked about the standard professional and academic criteria for choice of research problems, and about the mandate to publish (given the nonprofit public-domain nature of the foundation), no matter which interests might be offended. Blandy assented, with no equivocation. I then asked if I could have an annual seed-money fund of $10,000 or so, to parcel out to graduate students all over the country who were working on dissertations related to the foundation's mission. He thought that was a good idea and readily agreed to it, too. I was completely disarmed and felt a bit silly about my preconceptions of the foundation.

Blandy asked me—if I was willing to be made an offer—what salary I would want and when I could start. I replied that I had little idea of the salary structure of the current foundation staff. He said that he was thinking of a salary between $12,000 and $15,000, plus fringes, like pension and health insurance. I remarked that, even for New York at that time, the salary range was quite generous. But what about expenses for visitors' lunches and travel? He said that all on-the-job expenses were covered; I should expect to travel, visit innovative medical care settings, attend professional meetings, and so on.

"When could you come?" Blandy asked.

"When do you want me?"

The answer was October 1. This was June. I said that I had several things to clear up in my current position. I did not want to leave anything to encumber Hobbs and his staff. I suggested that I come on October 1 and spend alternate weeks in New York and Ontario until January 1, 1953, with all expenses paid by the foundation. He agreed with no hesitation.

I had nothing left to bargain for; all my conditions had been met. I went back to Ontario to wait for a formal letter. It arrived shortly, with all the specifications discussed and an offer of $15,000, which tripled my current income. I wrote a letter of acceptance and asked if my moving expenses would be paid, an item I had overlooked. A return letter said, "Of course."

6

The Health
Information Foundation,
1952-1962

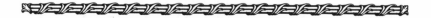

The idea of working for a foundation funded directly by a politically conservative industry, filtered through a board of directors made up of presidents of the major firms in drugs, pharmaceuticals, and chemicals, continued to worry me. I believed that Blandy and Williamson were honest and sincere and understood the mission of the foundation. I was ideally suited to the position, given my academic experience and my applied social research interests, and no questions were raised about my political orientation, liberal or conservative. This was during a period when academics, politicians, policymakers, the health professions, and insurance agencies took sides, and McCarthyism poisoned the political atmosphere. The debates at the time were so venomous that if I had still been on Sinai's staff when Admiral Blandy and Kenneth Williamson were looking for a research director, I might not have been considered because of my association with him.

Williamson, in a letter to me dated June 9, 1988, wrote that when the foundation was seeking names, he contacted heads of several departments of sociology, public-opinion people, directors of several foundations financing research, deans of several medical schools, and directors of the National Institutes of Health: "Out of all this we got three names, but Odin Anderson led all the rest." After I arrived at the foundation, Williamson told me that he had talked with the director of economic research at the American Medical Association, Frank Dickinson, about me. Dickinson, whom I knew well, said, "Odin is a good man, but watch him—he is too honest."

I had kept a low profile on advocacy but a high profile on producing data for policymaking in the American liberal-democratic range of politically feasible action. Some people may feel that this stance was evading the issues. I believed, however, that the foundation had the promise, through me, of contributing to a more rational discussion and debate in the controversial health services field. The foundation already had the financial resources for such an ambitious objective. I made a private decision to see what could be done in three years, and if I could not succeed, I would hope to be able to return to a more secure academic position. I had resigned from two such positions already. Health services research and medical sociology did not yet have a good base in universities.

The origin of the Health Information Foundation needs to be presented in some detail, to provide as clear a context as possible for the planning and operating base that I became a part of, and to develop an understanding of the research program concerned with health care policy issues in the United States. The idea of a foundation for educational and research purposes, financed by private money, is a characteristically American concept, mixing self-serving and genuinely altruistic motives difficult to unscramble. The same can be said, of course, for publicly financed endeavors for similar purposes. The letter from Williamson, already cited, has been most helpful, as have many conversations I had with him for the two years or so that we were together in the foundation.

For several years in the 1940s, the drug, pharmaceutical, and chemical industries had been helping to finance an effort, associated with the American Medical Association (AMA), to "expose the evils of socialized medicine." The details of this relationship between the industries named and the AMA are not known, at least not according to records. Naturally, the goodwill of the physicians was very important to these industries. The people directing the promotional literature against government health insurance made a critical mistake, however. Some of the promotional material sent to physicians was addressed "Dear Christian Doctor." The propaganda leaflets were also wrapped around the prescription bottles dispensed by pharmacists to patients. The first tactic was, of course, in very bad taste; the second evoked boycotts of pharmacies by labor unions in Cleveland and Minneapolis. The pharmacists hardly even knew what they were wrapping around the prescription bottles, and there was consternation on their part at the results. These methods made for dissatisfaction in the pharmaceutical industry, and it withdrew its financial support. The industry agreed with the objectives, but the methods being used tarnished its public image.

The upshot was that concerned leaders in the drug, pharmaceutical, and chemical industries felt that there was a need to do something constructive to inform the public about the strengths as well as the weaknesses of health care in this country, particularly the strengths. The major firms from which this leadership came were Searle Drug, Johnson & Johnson, Eli Lilly, Owens-Corning Glass, Sharpe and Dohme, Merck, S. B. Penick, American Home Products, American Hospital Supply, and others that Williamson could not recall in his letter to me. One member of this group, Bud Dempsey, president of Sharpe and Dohme, was very close to Stanley Resor, president and chairman of the J. Walter Thompson Company, a well-known public relations and advertising firm in New York (in fact, it was one of the three major firms of its kind).

Dempsey aroused the interest of Resor, and the involvement of the J. Walter Thompson agency followed. This agency had its headquarters in the centrally situated Graybar Building, adjoining Grand Central Station through a spacious corridor on the first floor, giving access to all the elevators to all floors in that office building. The public relations and advertising thrust for the future foundation was implicit but hardly spelled out. Its name, Health Information Foundation, its broad function, and its approach were developed with a small group of financial sponsors from the industries mentioned, under the guidance of Resor and his staff. The foundation was chartered in Illinois. The legal work was done by Norman Pritchard, partner in a prominent legal firm in Chicago.

It is pertinent to note that the pharmaceutical industry was a growth industry during this period after World War II. Its greatest growth was in antibiotics, which were very effective and gained wide publicity. There was thus a fair amount of discretionary money, which the presidents of the many large firms could use for what they regarded as worthy purposes. The Health Information Foundation was a clear example. Sums of $15,000 to $50,000 per firm quickly added up to around $500,000 a year. A rough measure of the growth was the value of pharmaceutical shipments from the industry. In 1947, for example, the total value was $941 million. By 1958, the total value was $2.6 billion. Inflation at that time was also minimal (U.S. Bureau of the Census, 1961).

After the foundation was chartered, the organizing group invited representatives of the medical and hospital organizations and the health insurance agencies to a meeting, where its purpose and financial support were outlined. A representative from the American Hospital Association was C. J. Foley, in charge of public relations. Comments and suggestions were sought. The organizing group planned to interest a nationally known person in becoming president of the foundation. This person was not to be drawn from the health field or even to have much knowledge of health affairs. The prominent one among several mentioned was Admiral Blandy. His name was put forward by Stanley Resor, who presented a very extensive background on him. Blandy was retiring as commander of the Atlantic fleet when he was officially approached about becoming president of the Health Information Foundation. Blandy symbolized patriotism and Americanism, but he was no jingoist.

The other matter discussed at this meeting was the need to employ a top assistant to Blandy, who would serve as executive vice-president. This person, however, was to be knowledgeable and experienced in the health field and guide the development of the foundation's program. C. J. Foley suggested to Kenneth Williamson, then on the administrative staff of the American Hospital Association, that Williamson apply for the job. The organizing group was to meet again, and Williamson attended. At this meeting, Williamson met Jack Searle, president of Searle Drug, and the others. Williamson told Searle he was interested in the job, and Searle requested a letter expressing interest. Williamson drew on his extensive contacts, such as Foster McGaw, chairman of American Hospital Supply and a close friend of Searle. McGaw contacted Searle and George Smith of Johnson & Johnson in support. George Bugbee, then executive director of the American Hospital Association, also wrote a letter to Searle, recommending Williamson.

Shortly thereafter, Williamson was offered the job and was told that Blandy would be president. Williamson requested of Searle that he be able to meet Blandy before he committed himself. Williamson met with Searle and Blandy jointly. Williamson writes: "Blandy was an impressive person and he seemed to be a very decent fellow. However, it was very apparent to me that he was very used to being 'in command' and he had lots to learn about civilian life and about voluntarism in the voluntary health field. There is very little 'commanding' that goes on." Williamson reports that Blandy really struggled with the slow pace of "willingness to cooperate" and learned that he was "very smart, a really fine person."

Space was obtained in the Graybar Building. Staff needs were discussed, and Williamson set about hiring supporting personnel. Since Blandy did not know people in the health or foundation field, Williamson arranged meetings with all such people. The board of the foundation did not want a tie with the AMA, although it thought that good relations should be cultivated. Very early on, Blandy moved to give the foundation a broad public image by appointing an advisory group of leading public figures. Through his friendship with ex-president Herbert Hoover, Blandy persuaded Hoover to be the chairman of the Citizens Advisory Group. Eventual members of this group were Donald Douglas, president of Douglas Aircraft; Dr. Lee A. DuBridge, president of California Institute of Technology, who had been a classmate of Blandy at Annapolis; Lewis L. Strauss, a key figure on Wall Street, whom President Eisenhower appointed to his cabinet; Dr. Karl T. Compton, chairman of the corporation, Massachusetts Institute of Technology; Ferdinand Eberstadt, president of F. Eberstadt and Company; Mrs. Oscar A. Ahlgren, president, General Federation of Women's Clubs; Allan B. Kline, president, American Farm Bureau Federation; and Dr. Franklyn B. Snyder, president emeritus, Northwestern University. This advisory group was assured that the foundation was no gimmick to promote drugs and sundries but was to be a high-level public service. Williamson reported that Blandy sent the members of the Citizens Advisory Group material and messages about the foundation, but he never had them "do anything" and was probably assured that they would not be expected to. They served a good purpose in itself, by helping to give the foundation a favorable and prestigious public image.

Williamson observed that the board of the foundation had a belief, bordering on a creed, that an informed public would act wisely and properly regarding health care policy. The foundation was to gather facts and information through its own staff, by making grants to researchers in universities, and by publicizing facts and information. All channels of communication would be used—research reports, books, and mass media. The J. Walter Thompson agency had assumed that it would supply the staff. In a short time, however, Williamson concluded that this arrangement was not workable; the foundation would need its own core research staff. Resor, of J. W. Thompson, was advising that research projects be directed to traditional public health problems, like health education, preventive medicine, and similar relatively noncontroversial areas. Williamson was aware that, so far, public health had done little or nothing about medical care organization and finance or about health insurance—in short, about problems of health services delivery or how communities develop health policy. In due course, the foundation and the Thompson agency parted company. Williamson and Blandy formulated their own policy for research and dissemination and presented it to the board by the end of the 1950s. It was accepted readily.

A young Ph.D. in sociology from Michigan State University, Walter Boek, was hired as a research analyst. A Ph.D. student in sociology from Columbia University, Patrick Murphy, was hired as his assistant. Three community health policy decision-making studies were contracted for with the sociology departments at Michigan State University, the University of North Carolina, and the University of Alabama. A grant was made to the Department of Sociology at Wayne State University, to study the public relations program of the Toledo (Ohio) Academy of Medicine. Also in progress was a project with Oscar Serbein, an economist at Columbia University, to write a sourcebook on voluntary health insurance and other methods to pay for health services. An annual directory of social research in the health services was compiled and disseminated to the academic social science research community. Questionnaires were sent to all social science departments and schools of public health in the country, querying what was in progress in health services research. This directory made for great visibility in the academic community.

On the mass-media side, the foundation, with its public re-

lations director, Edward Leibert, commissioned audiovisual experts
to create glossy television and cinema spots on activities in the
country related to research and accomplishments in medicine. By
early 1952, it turned out that these worthy activities were not making any splashes. Further, the research analyst and Williamson were
not seeing eye to eye on what research to promote. Williamson was
hoping to do a national household survey—"who gets what when
and where for how much"—on expenditures for personal health
services; a consumer survey; and a survey on how voluntary health
insurance, by the early 1950s, was helping households pay for expensive medical episodes. The research analyst warned Williamson
that such projects would be much too controversial for the conservative sponsors funding the foundation. Williamson was a risk
taker. The research analyst had a weak title and a weak position in
the foundation. He was young and inexperienced. He was, in part,
a victim of a relatively formless objective and policy, which he could
not be expected to transcend. He was dismissed. The foundation
was going through a traumatic learning process. It was spending
far more of its annual budget of $500,000 on the media than on
research, which was to be the source of solid information for media
dissemination. More time was needed for research—which, of
course, takes time. The board was impatient for rapid visibility of
the foundation.

Williamson and Blandy decided, during this seeming impo-
tence of the foundation, to attract a relatively senior researcher, with
standing and accomplishments in health services research, who
would have the title of research director. That is when I came in,
to great expectations of me and solid backing for whatever I might
decide should be the content of the research program, through research with my own staff and grants to universities—and enough
research money at hand for me to plan big and meet reasonable
deadlines. In a short time, most of the annual budget was allocated
to me, rather than to public relations. As it happened, I arrived and
started full-time work on October 1, 1952, for I had managed to
complete and write up the projects I had started at the University
of Western Ontario.

My Introduction to the Foundation

At the age of thirty-eight, which is not young, I felt a heavy responsibility in an environment rather different from my familiar academic one, which had been the setting for my entire professional life of twelve years. There was money, and action was expected. I had to test the promises that Blandy and Williamson had made: that the foundation was to be objective and in the public domain, a professional organization with academic standards. I had to have faith that the board had the same views.

As a New Deal liberal, I harbored the usual stereotypical image of big business as being very conservative on social issues. In the health field, I was part of the group of people in the Section on Medical Care of the American Public Health Association that, together with the association, was annually advocating a comprehensive federal-state national health insurance plan, central and local planning, group practice, and salaried physicians—in short, an ideological blueprint. Many of the advocates were "young turk" physicians with whom I had become friendly and who respected my work with Sinai. Temperamentally and pragmatically, I never shared their (to my mind) quite utopian plans. I shared Sinai's pragmatism about what was possible, and they were even critical of his pragmatic approach. In any case, I was regarded as "one of them," although somewhat on the fringes. I was producing research that they found useful for their policy advocacy.

In November 1952, six weeks after I arrived in New York to take the new job, I attended the annual meeting of the American Public Health Association in Cleveland, Ohio. By this time, my public health colleagues knew about my appointment, and I sensed some mixed feelings about the propriety of a person like me, with liberal leanings, going to work for an agency sponsored by a politically conservative industry, which was on record as being opposed to national health insurance. This attitude toward me was expressed very sharply at the association meeting, where I attended the annual meeting of the Group Health Association of America (GHAA), a federation of group-practice prepayment plans, and a struggling organization at that time, for there were not many such plans in existence. The meeting had been announced in the program as an open meeting, and so, with a Canadian health economist, I decided to attend and learn what was going on. In fact, I knew almost all of the representatives of the plans attending.

The meeting was about to start when my Canadian colleague and I walked in and sat down. The president at that time was Fred Mott, who was chairing the meeting. We knew each other very well. Mott was a U.S. citizen, trained in medicine at McGill University, in Montreal. Before directing a provincewide hospital insurance plan in Saskatchewan, he had been head of the much touted United Mine Workers "model" medical plan, financed by a surtax on coal. Mott was steeped in the group-practice prepayment idea. When he saw me come in and sit down, he strode quickly over to me and, with no preliminary warning, said, "Odin, given your new position, you do not belong here. Get out." Thunderstruck, my Canadian colleague and I walked out. I did sense some commotion in the assembled group of around thirty people.

Shortly after I returned to New York, I had a telephone call from Dr. Morris Brand, who was the medical director of the Sidney Hillman Health Center in New York, and whom I had gotten to know.

"Odin, what happened in Cleveland with Fred Mott?" he wanted to know.

I told him.

He said, "This is outrageous. I am the next president of the GHAA, and I extend a personal invitation to attend the next annual meeting."

Michael M. Davis, a well-known consultant, not-so-gray eminence, and lobbyist for national health insurance, called me from Washington, D.C., and asked what had gone on in Cleveland. I told him, and he also said, in effect, that Mott's action was outrageous. I had met Davis before, when I worked with Sinai. I saw him many times later on in Washington. Thereafter, I had brief problems with both liberals and conservatives, which I will describe later.

Developing a Research Program

Fortunately, when I arrived, Williamson had already started discussions with Clyde Hart, director of the National Opinion Research Center, University of Chicago, for a nationwide household survey of health services expenditures and voluntary health insurance. No such survey had been conducted since CCMC's report, in 1933. The timing for another nationwide survey was perfect. President Truman's departure from the White House, and the installation of Dwight D. Eisenhower as the first Republican president since 1933, created a political calmness around the question of government health insurance, in contrast to the strident days of Truman. A major disappointment for Truman was that he had not succeeded in convincing Congress to enact national health legislation. In fact, the very commission that Truman appointed, the President's Commission for the Health Needs of the Nation, sidestepped the issue and left the field open to continued growth of voluntary health insurance to solve the problems of insurance for at least the majority of the American public. Voluntary health insurance, in 1952, was covering over 50 percent of the population, an achievement that exceeded even the expectations of its proponents. In this atmosphere, it became opportune and feasible to float a national health survey to find out about consumers' problems with current expenditures for health services and the extent to which voluntary health insurance was helping households.

Williamson wondered what I would think of backing this household survey. It was made to order for me, in terms of my interests, my experience, the proper timing, and my tutelage under Nathan Sinai. I believed that if we could get the board's approval for such a bold and expensive project (for that time), it would in itself be worth my move to the Health Information Foundation. The board members, all presidents of major drug firms, seemed to carry over to the foundation their experience with research in the drug, pharmaceutical, and chemical firms. They had respect for research as such, although social research was new to them. The research already completed or in progress at the foundation when I arrived was relatively cheap—$10,000 here, $25,000 there, and so on. What Williamson and I were proposing was in the $250,000 range for one major effort—the entire research budget for that year, at one crack.

I immediately started to work with the National Opinion Research Center (NORC) on planning and designing the first household survey of its kind since 1933. We had a marvelous collegial relationship. I was responsible for the content of the questionnaire for personal household interviews. NORC counseled me on the feasibility of acquiring the information desired from informants, the size of the sample, how it would be drawn, and other such details. We also proposed a survey of two cities, to compare the efficacy of Blue Cross–Blue Shield plans in one and a mainline private insurance plan in the other. Between October 1 and December 1, 1952, we fashioned a complete research proposal, with budget and deadlines, for my first meeting with the board. The meeting was held on December 1, 1952, at the University Club on Fifth Avenue, the usual meeting place. We started with lunch, where Clyde Hart was present to answer questions. How would this survey assist in the expansion of voluntary health insurance? The answer was that voluntary health insurance would use the data, particularly the Blue Cross–Blue Shield plans. Would this proposed survey duplicate any other surveys under way in the country? The answer was no. One board member remarked that we should help President Eisenhower to meet the needs of low-income groups, in connection with legislation that his administration might sponsor.

Clyde Hart left after lunch, and we went into executive session. Jack Searle was the chairman. After less than ten minutes of discussion (apparently, the board members had read the proposal in advance), Searle said, "Well, gentlemen, this looks like a good project. Let us pass it with a show of hands." It was unanimous. In that short time, the board approved the research proposal and a budget of $275,000 (in 1952 dollars), $200,000 for NORC and $75,000 for the research director's expenses (Health Information Foundation, 1952). Searle remarked that he had not expected social research to be so expensive, but he did not flinch. He was used to spending millions of dollars on pharmaceutical research. NORC promised to have preliminary results by the end of 1953 or early 1954—a staggering promise, given the complicated operational logistics of social surveys. I left the meeting overwhelmed by the responsibility that NORC and I had assumed.

The next meeting was on February 3, 1953. During the interim, Searle and the board had become impatient. They now asked Hart, who again was present, if the project could be speeded up.

Hart said this could be done for another $35,000, which the board immediately approved. Preliminary results were to be available in November 1953. The first full draft of findings would be ready by March 1, 1954, and the final report would be finished by June 1, 1954, to be followed by a book and survey methodology, to be published as soon as possible (Health Information Foundation, 1953).

I flew or took the overnight train from New York to NORC in Chicago about once a month, to work with the staff until the field phase and preliminary tabulations were completed (basically on time). The interval between the approval of the project and the preliminary data gave me time to work up other ideas for future projects. It was the policy of the board that the money the industry contributed annually was not to be accumulated and left unused. The foundation was to maintain a momentum of overlapping projects. The funding momentum from the industry was such that it could commit funds for projects in advance of money in reserve. I had the impression that I could propose and start projects on a three-year lead time, knowing that the industry, through the board, would maintain the funding momentum that far ahead. This meant that I could hire and hold staff from project to project, even keeping one on salary who was not on a project but could be used for data gathering in one area or another. For an academician, the pace was dizzy but manageable.

While the nationwide survey was in the field, I began to formulate another major project: to study the operation of the medical prepayment plans in Windsor, Ontario, and the county medical bureaus owned by the county medical societies in the state of Washington. It will be recalled that I had become very familiar with both sites while on Sinai's staff at the University of Michigan, and I was well known in both places. As I was formulating my research philosophy and strategy in relation to the current controversies over different types of delivery systems, I decided that the most logical and legitimate strategy was, for the time being, to evaluate the existing and prevailing voluntary health insurance systems—at that time, the group-practice prepayment types of health insurance, with salaried physicians, a known population paying monthly premiums from their own pockets or with the help of employers, and no charges (to speak of) at time of service. In some instances, these plans owned their own hospitals or contracted with hospitals in the community. The well-known ones—practically the only ones at that time—were Group Health in Washington, D.C., Group Health in Seattle, Kaiser Permanente on the West Coast, and the Health Insurance Plan of Greater New York. The mainstream medical associations fought these plans vigorously as intrusions into the mainstream fee-for-service arrangement. The plans' growth was hampered by this opposition because it was difficult to recruit physicians in such a hostile atmosphere.

The prevailing voluntary health insurance pattern at this time was Blue Cross for hospital care, Blue Shield for physicians' services, and private insurance companies for both. Their strength in marketing was the prevailing structure of practice, to which people were accustomed. Their weakness, for insurance purposes, was the lack of coverage for home and office calls, which they feared were financially uncontrollable. Physicians' services were limited to in-hospital surgery and whatever nonsurgical care was judged to require the patient to be in a hospital. Windsor and the state of Washington had been demonstrating for a dozen years that home and office calls were feasible to cover, but mainstream medicine in general did not believe this and stuck to the limited Blue Shield plans and private insurance companies. I thought that if the basis of the controversy was lack of information, rather than ideology, perhaps controversy could be reduced by facts. I felt that mainstream medicine should be more aware that these comprehensive fee-for-service plans worked and could be a reasonable compromise to adopt, simply by expanding the Blue Shield plans to home and office calls. There were ideologists on both sides, in mainstream medicine and among the proponents of group-practice prepayment. The latter thought that mainstream health insurance, with fee-for-service, was inefficient and costly and did not stress prevention. I proposed to Williamson and Blandy that we explore this "middle way" by contracting with Nathan Sinai's Bureau of Public Health Economics at the University of Michigan to study these two plans. By this time, Sinai had quite an adequate staff and would be able to move quickly.

Here, I took a calculated risk, which would test the board, accomplish a legitimate policy research objective, and be a token of appreciation for Sinai for having inducted me into this fascinating research field. The risk entailed contracting with Sinai, given his persona non grata status in mainstream medicine. Sinai's group was then the best-qualified academic research unit to conduct a study of this nature. Williamson and Blandy agreed readily to this proposal.

The proposal was brought up for discussion on January 7, 1954. It was discussed at length and held in abeyance. It was approved in principle but turned over to the Operating Committee (whose function I did not fully understand) for further consideration, to be brought up at a future meeting of the board. I recall Blandy's disappointment as we were walking back to the office. He was not used to being delayed and possibly turned down. He said, "We will beat them next time."

In the meantime, to return to the progress of the national household survey, I reported at the regular meeting of the board on September 14, 1953, that the preliminary tabulations would be available in November 1953, as promised. This news prompted one board member to reveal that the Senate Committee on Labor and Public Welfare had been made aware of the forthcoming data and requested access to it. An editorial review board, to go over my report with me, was to be appointed and selected from among technical advisers and the industry. The industry reviewers turned out to be research scientists and were very cooperative.

My three regular technical advisers were Louis Dublin, formerly a well-known statistician, retired from the Metropolitan Life Insurance Company and past president of the American Public Health Association; C. Rufus Rorem, chairman of the Hospital Council in Philadelphia and active in the start of the Blue Cross plans, with a Ph.D. in economics from the University of Chicago; and Franz Goldman, associate professor of public health, Yale University, formerly in the top hierarchy of public health in Hitler's Germany, from which he had fled. Dublin had already been appointed when I arrived at the foundation, and I was asked to name two more consultants. I chose Rorem because he had wide connections in Blue Cross plans and hospitals. Goldman I chose because he had connections in the group-health movement. They were put on an annual retainer. They proved very useful in helping to legitimate me as a researcher with their respective constituencies. They were, of course, helpful in occasional individual discussions on the health field generally.

They were widely different personalities. Dublin was pompous and felt he was all-knowing, but he did know a lot. I recall his very first visit. He sat down in front of my desk and asked, "Well, Odin, what do you want to know?" No discussion. Rorem would come in, sit in front of my desk, and ask, "Well, Odin, what ideas can we put on the table to discuss today?" Goldman would come in and sit in the same position, but at the first meeting, he asked if he could get a grant to study long-term care in general hospitals— an inappropriate request, given his role. He was very helpful and sympathetic with my position, and I was a frequent dinner guest at his home in New Haven, as I was at Rorem's in Philadelphia.

Excitement was gathering for the release of the preliminary data on the national survey, now set for a press conference in New York on January 18, 1954. NORC fed me table after table from Chicago, which I put together in a preliminary format by January 14. The foundation's director of public relations, Ed Leibert, was waiting patiently enough to get the report in time to prepare a news release and organize the press conference. My report had to be reviewed collegially by the staff of NORC in Chicago before it was released. I took the typewritten report to Chicago on an overnight train. I spent the day with NORC, cleared all details, and took the overnight train back to New York, arriving at the foundation office in the early forenoon. Leibert was at the door, literally grabbing the report from my hands. I told him, as a researcher, that my reputation and that of NORC for validity and accuracy was at stake, whereas, when his job was completed, the press release would vanish into thin air. I should add, however, that he was very good to work with. We played our roles. We were all geared up for this publicity event.

Then, suddenly, Admiral Blandy died at home from a stroke while sitting at his desk, on January 12. The press conference was postponed from January 18 to January 19. I had a meeting with my review committee the day after Blandy's death. The committee was very satisfied with my report; no changes were suggested at all.

The date for the press conference was timed so that the newspapers could have several days to prepare articles for the Sunday editions. The press conference was well attended. With the NORC staff, I gave a short report after handing out press releases. The newspapers' interest was great. Questions were for clarification. I recall that Earl Ubell, science writer for the *New York Herald Tribune*, asked me how the sample was drawn. "It is an area probability sample . . . ," I began. He cut me short. "That's good enough for me," he said. I was no sampling expert, and I was glad I could pronounce the name of the sampling method correctly. After I went home to Westchester for dinner, I had a call from the *New York Times* reporter. He said that his editor was not satisfied with the percentages I gave for the composition of the medical dollar (hospitals, physicians, dentists, and so on), which added up to 101 percent. Could I give the exact percentages, to the first decimal point? I did, but I also told him that degree of specificity was not necessary for the purpose.

That Sunday, all the major newspapers in the country, from coast to coast, prominently carried the story on the results of the household survey: average annual expenditure per household for health services, including drugs; percentage covered by voluntary health insurance; how many people were in debt for health services, above a certain amount. This last item was played up, to the rumored discomfiture of the board. Williamson and I crowed that the board got the visibility it had wanted, and more. We became nationally known that weekend, and the board was pleased but nervous.

A New President

On January 18, 1954, the board met in emergency session, six days after Blandy's death and a few hours after his funeral, which the members had attended in Washington, D.C. The admiral was buried with full military honors in Arlington Cemetery.

I did not attend the funeral or the board meeting. Williamson did. To add to the tension for me, Williamson had resigned from the foundation shortly before the admiral's death, to become director of the Washington office of the American Hospital Association. He agreed with the board to shuttle between Washington and New

York to help run the foundation until successors could be found for both him and Blandy. Williamson reported that there was no hesitation on the part of the board about continuing the foundation. It unanimously moved immediately to find a successor to Blandy as president of the foundation. This time, the board would search for a person who knew the health field and was well connected professionally in it. Several names were mentioned, including that of George Bugbee, who was then executive director of the American Hospital Association.

In his autobiography, Bugbee writes that early in 1954 he was approached by J. D. Searle, chairman of the foundation's board. Searle asked Bugbee if he could be persuaded to become president. Searle, knowing Bugbee's personal circumstances, asked if he would like to spend his summers at Genesee Depot, Wisconsin, not far from Milwaukee, where he had a comfortable summer home on the eighty-acre estate owned by his brother-in-law, the actor Alfred Lunt, and Lunt's wife, the actress Lynn Fontanne. Bugbee could operate the foundation from there. Bugbee wrote, "This provided a base from which I might affect health policy, my most interesting . . . activity" (Bugbee, 1987, p. 128). He recognized the possibly self-serving aspects of the sponsors but was in general agreement with their objectives.

Bugbee assumed the presidency of the Health Information Foundation on May 1, 1954. He was a perfect choice for that position. He was highly respected in the health services field as a professional administrator and health policymaker, but he had always kept a low profile. He was a graduate (in accounting) of the School of Business of the University of Michigan. His career, up to this appointment, included being an accountant at the University Hospital of the University of Michigan in 1926 and rising to assistant director. In 1938, he became superintendent of the Cleveland City Hospitals, until 1943. In that year, he became executive director of the American Hospital Association. During that eleven-year period, Bugbee built the association up to a prominent position in health services. His major influence on health policy at that time was his role in the formulation of the Hospital Survey and Construction Act, passed with support of all interest groups in 1946. The act was designed to improve and expand the hospitals of this country after

World War II. The war had suspended the building, improvement, and distribution of hospitals. The method was to use federal start-up costs, through state plans, matched by local hospitals (a one-shot subsidy).

It is obvious that Bugbee's background and interests were ideal for the foundation. What was further revealed as very salutory for the foundation's mission was Bugbee's view that the health field needed more information for rational policymaking and for teaching content in the rapidly growing programs in health services administration in universities. It would seem that the Bugbee-Anderson combination would be a unique one, given the objective of social research related to public policy. Bugbee had the constituency of the health services provider infrastructure to which to direct research results. I had access to the health services research emerging infrastructure. We combined a working knowledge of the nature of the health services delivery system(s) and the American political process. We had symbiotic skills and differential rewards—Bugbee, as president, relating to the daily working world through contacts and occasional speeches, and myself relating to the research world. We were not so far apart politically that we were unable to work together ideologically. We both accepted the liberal-democratic political model, Bugbee toward the conservative pole and myself toward the American liberal pole, but we were both within the vital center of those poles. We discussed health policy frequently, but our ideological differences were a matter of degree and could be negotiated, as it were, through political-process compromises. Our relationship was an ideal one for the purposes of the foundation's mission.

A couple of months before Bugbee formally took over the presidency of the foundation, he visited the foundation so that I could brief him on the current status of our research program and the planning for it. He asked me, "Odin, are you treading water? Do any decisions need to be made before I start, so that you are not held back but can maintain momentum?" I said no; we had enough going on to keep us busy until he arrived, after which we could go on from there.

During the interim between Admiral Blandy's death and Bugbee's arrival, the board had approved the project with Sinai's research unit in the School of Public Health at the University of Michigan. The project was split into two parts and two contracts. The Windsor, Ontario, part of the project was under contract when Bugbee took over. The Washington State part was still in negotiation among Sinai, the Washington medical bureaus, and the foundation. Sinai needed time to explore the State of Washington's situation in terms of the setting and the likely degree of cooperation before he and his staff could design a proposal for costs, time, and scope. I also had another project in progress, on the organizational and technical problems of Blue Cross and Blue Shield in enrolling members who were not in employed groups (the usual enrollment technique). Could self-employed farmers and others be formed into groups? I hired a sociologist, Sol Levine, to head that project.

At the first executive committee meeting of the board in which Bugbee participated, it was reported that there were relationship problems developing regarding the personnel and the agency involved in conducting these studies. It turned out that unidentified physicians (at least not identified to me or to Bugbee) had been calling board members and telling them that Sinai was not acceptable because of his having been a consultant to California's Governor Earl Warren in formulating a state health insurance program in the 1940s; he had even testified for it before a state legislative committee. I was exceedingly sorry that this was the first (and potentially messy) order of business that Bugbee had to deal with after occupying his position. I did not attend the meeting, but Bugbee transmitted the discussion to me in some detail. In addition, he seemed to be rather calm and collected about what I regarded as a crisis for us and the foundation and its future. As I said earlier, I had taken a calculated risk on Sinai's reputation with some of the leaders in the medical profession, although I gathered that his reputation for solid research was not in question. The executive committee agreed that the chairman of the board and Bugbee should explore this problem further. I had already been out to the state of Washington to explore the possibilities for doing a study there and was favorably received by medical bureau leaders, who remembered me from my previous fieldwork there.

Perhaps I overreacted (unlike Bugbee), although I tried to be as calm and collected as he was, but I felt that a crisis of principles was looming, and I visualized the possibility of the executive committee's demanding that we break our contracts with Sinai, the Windsor project, and Washington. I called my staff together and informed them of this critical situation and said that if the executive committee broke the Windsor contract, I would resign. (I was opposed to stopping the medical bureau project as well, but, technically, it was not yet under contract.) I never told Bugbee about this staff meeting or my possible action. Bugbee conferred with Sinai in Ann Arbor by telephone and immediately left to discuss with him how to handle the Windsor and Washington State projects.

When Bugbee returned from Ann Arbor he said little about the atmosphere in which he and Sinai came to their mutual agreements, describing the uproar in the board as a tempest in a teapot. One of Sinai's senior staff members, Solomon Axelrod, reported to me that the discussion and negotiations were very professional and candid; he was most impressed. The result was that Sinai would retain the Windsor project in Ontario, an area in which he was not at all controversial. He would withdraw from further pursuit of the Washington medical bureau project; there was an implied commitment but no contract.

Accelerated Research and Publicity

The foundation's and the board's interest in the medical bureau project continued unabated. The financial appropriation for it had already been made, pending a final proposal. How to go on from there? During my two summers, 1945 and 1947, doing field research in the state of Washington, I had become well acquainted with George Shipman, a professor of political science who had a good grasp of and interest in the health and public welfare activities of the state. I called him up and asked if I could fly out and talk with him about a project I had in mind. I did so, immediately after our agreement with Sinai.

I spent a couple of days with Shipman, telling him about the background and development with Sinai, and I said I was now free to discuss the possible interest Shipman might have in the project, as well as the resources of the University of Washington that he could put together. His interest was immediate, and he mentioned two potential collaborators: Robert Lampman, a professor of economics, and S. Frank Miyamoto, a professor of sociology. Shipman would confer with them and report back. I flew back to New York.

In a short time, he reported that this team was interested. I asked him to prepare a research proposal and a budget. Before long, the proposal was submitted and accepted, and a contract was made. This was in the latter part of 1954. The medical bureau leaders were willing to cooperate fully with the University of Washington team and me. To cap the relationship, I was invited by the Federation of County Medical Bureaus (of which there were twenty-one) to attend the annual meeting of the federation in Spokane, late in the fall of 1954, as the research project was getting under way, and address the meeting, describing and explaining the nature and scope of the project. Before that meeting, I was in Seattle (King County) to have a preliminary meeting with Dr. Shelby Jared, executive director of the King County Medical Bureau, who was then also president of the federation. He was exceedingly cordial, recalling times past. He said that I might expect some hostility and suspicion from the audience of physicians, but he would handle them. "You know how doctors are," he said.

This was, of course, a very crucial event for me. An entire project was at stake. It had more implications for health services delivery policy in the United States than the Windsor project did because Windsor's experience was not regarded as relevant to this country. A very personal aspect of this meeting is that I was replacing Nathan Sinai. I was trusted more than my own mentor, who had brought me into this field of research. I felt a keen sense of risk that I was implicitly repudiating Sinai in the role I was playing. Thirty-seven years later, I still vividly recall this feeling.

What to tell this audience? By this time, I had the data from the national household survey—to a great extent, the same type of information that would be collected on the medical bureaus' experience. Therefore, I extrapolated the national data to the population that the bureaus were covering and made rough estimates of the impact that the bureaus had on expenditures, both for in-hospital physicians' services and for home and office calls. (Mainstream health insurance outside the state of Washington was not covering home and office calls.) This strategy worked very well. The audience liked hard data. Several in the audience told me that they had never heard such a lucid presentation on the predicted operation of the medical bureaus. I flew back to New York quite content that the project was under control and that my relationship with Sinai was intact.

After the Sinai flurry, the foundation program moved ahead and took on, I believe, a research policy related to problems in the health services. Bugbee immediately narrowed the audience to which the publicity was directed, from a blanketing of fairly soft information for a mass audience to an audience of policymakers, administrators, bureaucrats, and health insurance agencies. The current director of public relations was released, and an editor and writer, Michael Lesparre, was hired to assist in the editing and publicity of the research results, which started to flow. Bugbee built the foundation activities around my research.

Out of an average annual budget of $500,000, $400,000 was allocated to research and publication costs. I gather that the board did set up some sort of publication-review committee before the research was published, but we never were asked to change anything. Later, even this procedure was abolished. Instead, before publication of any research, if we felt that there might be trouble because of certain findings or their interpretation, we warned the board members in advance, so that they would not be taken by surprise.

Shortly after Bugbee arrived, my staff and I, particularly Patrick Murphy, conceived of a monthly bulletin on various aspects of health and the health services, to be called *Progress in Health Services*. The first trial bulletin was a review of declining crude mortality in the United States from 1900 to 1954, age-specific and net improvements. With the help of Michael Lesparre, we put out a highly technical but still readable review, with colored charts. We mailed it free of charge to thousands of people in the health field and to the print media. It was an instant success. We followed up the first issue with issues on age at death in the United States, changes in leading causes of death, increasing life expectancy at birth, and our aging population (remember, this was thirty-seven years ago, before such data were systematically analyzed). Later, we drew on the national survey of households for our bulletin on what

Americans spend for personal health services. The latter issue was exceedingly popular.

In the middle of all this, Murphy died from an unremovable shrapnel wound in his spine, sustained in World War II. In a short time, I was able to attract Monroe Lerner, a Ph.D. student in demography at Columbia University and a staff member of the popular *Statistical Bulletin* of the Metropolitan Life Insurance Company. The *Bulletin* had been the brainchild of Louis Dublin many years earlier. From 1956 to 1962, we published ten monthly bulletins a year on a wide range of subjects, including an estimate of people without insurance.

With respect to my career, I worried about the break in continuity of my academic aspirations. Fortunately, Wellman Warner, then head of the Department of Sociology at New York University, and Henry Meyer, also a professor there, visited me in 1953 and asked if I would give a seminar for graduate students. (I had already hired one of their graduates, Sol Levine, who in turn hired Gerald Gordon, then a Ph.D. student. In fact, the Department of Sociology at New York University became my source of research assistants at the foundation for a number of projects. The foundation became like a graduate department in sociology, with a lively research component.) The idea was that I would conduct an evening seminar in the fall semester, once a week. Warner said candidly that he had no money to pay me, but perhaps having a continuing academic appointment as adjunct associate professor would be reward enough. He also said that my salary at the foundation was far above salaries paid to faculty at that time, which was true. Thus, one evening a week I took the subway down to Washington Square, had supper in Greenwich Village, and conducted the seminar. This was strenuous but very rewarding, both academically and in terms of the students I attracted. At least four of them are now well-known medical sociologists or in related research areas.

In 1956, I left New York University to accept an offer as adjunct associate professor in the School of Public Health and Administrative Medicine at Columbia University, until 1962. I did not give a course but gave occasional lectures on call. Unfortunately, I did not have any graduate students, given this arrangement, but I was back in a school of public health again. Ray Trussell was then dean and was very active in promoting research in the health services. He had policy connections with the state legislature. It was an interesting association for me in that I was able to observe the politics of policy research closely. I believe I was able thus to maintain a semblance, at least, of academic continuity, which probably helped in my move to the University of Chicago.

To return to the continuing development of the research program, social survey methodology and technology had, fortunately, reached a high degree of accuracy and validity, and I used it to the hilt in its application to the health field. The NORC staff and I gained a great deal of experience in survey problems peculiar to the health field (particularly the problem of informants' recall of their use of and expenditure for health services over various lengths of time) and in comparing informants' reports with hospital and physicians' records. Social surveys of this magnitude were not cheap. Fortunately, our research budgets were quite adequate, and the board did not stint on ensuring validity with adequate samples and personal interviews in homes, rather than on the telephone.

The first household survey, as already noted, was conducted in 1953–54. A book was published by McGraw-Hill in 1956. I wrote the text, and Jacob Feldman, my collaborating methodologist from NORC, wrote the methodology for the appendix (Anderson and Feldman, 1956). The publication was subsidized by the foundation. From 1954 to 1958, we mounted three more nationwide social surveys with NORC: on adults' recognition of symptoms that would reasonably require medical attention; on attitudes toward health and illness; and on attitudes toward physicians, nurses, hospitals, and related matters. Briefly, we found that the American public was quite sophisticated in its knowledge of symptoms. This study became useful for health educators. Feldman, the project director, was the author of the book on this study (Feldman, 1966). (The study became Feldman's dissertation for a Ph.D. in sociology at the University of Chicago. I was on his committee. I always tried to get some academic spinoffs from the foundation research.)

The second survey, in 1958, was a repeat of the first household survey on expenditures for and use of health services. It turned out that the health services field, at this time and later on as well, was so dynamic that a repeat of the 1953–54 survey was indicated.

The health field and government statistical agencies were clamor-
ing for updated information. It is of interest that the U.S. Public
Health Service and relevant federal agencies were reluctant to engage in the type of survey research we were promoting at the foundation because of its political sensitivity regarding the implications
for government and voluntary health insurance. In fact, the foundation data became the official data for health services use and
expenditures and for the performance of voluntary health insurance. These data were incorporated annually into federal reports. It
was only much later, in the 1960s, that the Bureau of the Census and
the new National Center for Health Statistics were able to collect
routinely the type of data we produced through the foundation. I
knew the government people well. They were glad that we were
producing such valuable data for public policy, data too "hot" to
be produced by a public agency. I thought such data production was
a legitimate public responsibility in a democracy, and that a private
agency should not be expected to assume this function indefinitely.
In time, the National Center for Health Statistics was established,
as the political atmosphere surrounding health insurance became
more congenial.

The second survey enabled us to monitor changing patterns
in the health services over a five-year period. Again, the foundation
received a great deal of favorable publicity (Anderson, Collette, and
Feldman, 1963). To overcome inherent time lags between the gathering of preliminary and final data and the publication of a book,
we issued preliminary reports two to three years ahead of time, in
our *Progress in Health Services* or in our research series, which I
started in 1957. We also published books. The board did not want
the data to gather dust in our office.

The third household survey, started in 1957, was directed at
a nationwide sample of people sixty-five years of age and older.
This survey was a response to the debate, raging at that time, on
universal health insurance for the elderly. There was a clamor for
data, beyond the many horror stories emanating from anecdotal
sources. We floated the first household survey on the health circumstances of the elderly, their level of independent living, incomes,
and health insurance. We engaged Ethel Shanas, a demographer
trained at the University of Chicago and on the staff of NORC, to

be the project director, with myself as principal investigator. This was, of course, a study with direct political implications for a salient political issue at that time. Voluntary health insurance for the elderly and retirees was clearly inadequate at that time, and the study gave some hard data on the problem.

As I moved into this study with Shanas and the NORC, I began to realize that I was overloaded, having authored two household surveys already, plus some monographs and articles. Fortunately, Shanas clearly showed a capacity and an enthusiasm for the project as it developed. I then asked her if she would take over the whole project, from design to a final report. She did, to my relief (Shanas, 1962). (Shanas eventually became a nationally and internationally known social gerontologist, engaging in cross-national research. She has occupied well-regarded faculty positions in academic institutions.) Again, we released preliminary data for early publication, which fed into the data resources on the debate regarding health insurance for the elderly. Shanas was in great demand as a speaker.

The foregoing activities would seem to indicate that the foundation was floating on a sea of acceptance of its mission and of the research flowing from that mission. In substance, I believe this was true. There was always a feeling of uneasiness among us that the AMA would like to undermine us. I believe, however, that the AMA's hierarchy was astute enough not to bother us directly, although there may have been idiosyncratic individuals on the AMA staff looking for occasions to lash out at us. One morning, I was perusing the *Journal of the American Medical Association,* the issue dated February 23, 1957. I was startled to see, on page 655, a full-page headline—"Anderson Versus the U.S. Department of Commerce"—followed by a two-page article by Frank Dickinson, economist and director of the Bureau of Medical Economics of the AMA, attacking the methodology and some conclusions of the first household survey. Dickinson was angry (his writing style showed it) that our book had shown that, for July 1952 through June 1953, expenditures for physicians' services accounted for 37 percent of all components of health services, and hospitals accounted for 20 percent. According to Dickinson, the Department of Commerce's estimate for 1952 on expenditures for physicians was 28 percent and for hospital expenditures 26 percent. What Dickinson had been glee-fully showing in previous releases was that hospitals were accounting for approximately the same percentage of the medical dollar as physicians were. He wished to minimize the role of physicians in generating what was even then the high cost of health services. (This seems like nitpicking, but those were nitpicking days.) We had no business, Dickinson wrote, to revise the estimates made by the Department of Commerce with its methodology, and which, over time (according to him), had become sacrosanct. (Feldman told me that in conferring with personnel in the Department of Commerce, he learned that they believed our estimates were closer to being correct than theirs were, because of our method of gathering information. In our table, Feldman produced half a page of fine print, showing how his estimates were made.) Dickinson went even farther afield: "It seems rather strange that this report of a research group supported by private corporations whose existence depends on their ability to show profits should contain such comments as follows. . . . The problem is one of spreading this cost [the $10.2 billion spent on personal consumption expenditures for medical care] over all families through insurance premiums." He also criticized our observation that premiums should be related to income (Dickinson, 1957).

When I showed this attack to George Bugbee, he remarked, in his usual understated style, "Well, this will not be a pleasant day." Our industry sponsors were under attack. Bugbee contacted George Lull, general manager of the AMA, asking about this full-page editorial attack. Lull, according to Bugbee, said, "Well, George, you should have seen the first draft." (The two Georges had known each other for a long time while Bugbee was executive director of the American Hospital Association.) Bugbee contacted Jack Searle and other board members, who (according to Bugbee) shrugged their shoulders and let it pass. This attack did not have the slightest effect on our research policy.

Bugbee did not tell me until after we moved to the University of Chicago in 1962 that his first order of business when he became president of the foundation was, at the request of the chairman of the board, to evaluate my political views: How liberal was I? Bugbee believed that some physicians were calling board members to undermine my credibility. I believe that Bugbee withheld this information so as not to worry me (I am a worrying sort). Bugbee's answer to the board was that I was regarded as an objective researcher.

To give some idea of my relationship to "liberals" and "conservatives," I was asked by the nominating committee of the Section on Medical Care of the American Public Health Association, of which I was a charter member, to be nominated as a candidate for membership on its council. I accepted, but after talking with Bugbee about it, I withdrew. That section was being watched by quite reactionary interests, and I thought that it would be the better part of prudence not to be that visible. I was active in the section generally. Perhaps I overreacted, but such was the atmosphere of the time.

Nathan Sinai saw the attack on me in the AMA's journal, and on March 1, 1957, he wrote me a letter: "In this I think there is a lesson—one that I hoped you'd never experience [as he had]. The field of work is controversial and that applies to all logic and facts that may be presented. Therefore, never over-value the trappings of acceptance and cordiality. [And I was so treated during my occasional visits to the AMA, particularly by Dickinson.] And never undervalue the likelihood of quick armed aggression and undeclared war." Dickinson and I never visited or wrote to each other again. I had known him since the Sinai days in Michigan.

I might say in passing, although I have no idea whether the board felt that way, that my reputation as a liberal gave the foundation more credibility in the health policy debate, where liberals dominated, than if I had had the reputation of being a conservative Republican. It is fun to speculate. The more research I did on the health services delivery systems, here and abroad, the more I was sobered about the profound difficulties of reforming this complicated institution toward greater and greater equity, not to mention quality. Knowledge of society and institutions in itself can result in a conservative stance, through this very realization about the art of the possible. I could be called, as I sometimes reluctantly characterize myself, an "empirical conservative": my research has frequently resulted in findings that I wish were not so.

To continue with the Dickinson affair, I told my research staff not to correspond with or see Dickinson without my knowledge and permission. Given his possible sources of data, they might do so. Dickinson had frequently sent me AMA reports, for example. I was very uneasy, maybe overreacting, about relationships of my staff and myself to the outside. One of my staff members, an economist (Dickinson also was an economist), disregarded my request. I dressed him down, but he did not share my sense of strategy. He made me uneasy. I finally dismissed him, the only time I have fired a research staff member among all the researchers I have hired. To this day, he does not really understand my uneasiness. What is mystifying is that he continues to be very cordial toward me.

The foundation and its work were rapidly getting increasing and favorable attention in the health care field, both in the working world and in academia. In 1957, the Health Insurance Plan (HIP) of Greater New York, a staff-model group-practice prepayment plan, approached me through its research unit to do a study of the results of its trying out a dual-choice method for enrolling employed groups in the New York area. Its usual enrollment philosophy had been to offer its plan to various employed groups on a take-it-or-leave-it basis: all employees should enroll, or else there would be no deal. HIP had been in existence since 1946 and had enrolled a fair share of the population in the metropolitan area, but its growth was slowing down. As is inevitable, employees wanted more choice of plans within the group. The Kaiser Permanente plan on the West Coast was already offering a dual-choice arrangement with Blue Cross–Blue Shield.

HIP had offered its own plan, and Group Health Insurance (GHI), a comprehensive plan (including house and office calls), was offering its plan to the same employed groups in three labor unions. GHI was a fee-for-service plan. It turned out that the employees split down the middle in choosing HIP or GHI. HIP was curious about why most, if not all, of the employees did not choose HIP over GHI. Group-practice plans had a very high opinion of themselves. They felt that theirs was the rational way to deliver services, for physicians as well as patients. Would the foundation finance the study, and would I be the principal investigator?

My colleagues in the research unit in HIP, Paul Densen and Sam Shapiro, were both seasoned and excellent health services researchers, having conducted and published pertinent research on HIP performance. I jumped at this opportunity and engaged the

NORC office in New York, under Paul B. Sheatsley, to do the field survey. I said I would be pleased to do this project, if I could expand it from attitudes to utilization and cost patterns. This was agreed to.

One quite unexpected finding was that the GHI members were more satisfied with their plan than the HIP members were with theirs. Less surprising was that HIP members utilized hospital days and surgery considerably less than GHI members did. HIP was distressed by the attitudes but pleased with the lower utilization. HIP believed that its utilization was more "rational" and efficient than GHI's. Among HIP members, 79 percent were entirely and fairly well satisfied; among GHI members, 90 percent were entirely and fairly well satisfied. Twelve percent of the HIP members and 3 percent of the GHI members were dissatisfied. There were more details, but the foregoing differences may be sufficient for our purposes here. HIP was quite startled by the differences in satisfaction, and the HIP physicians were unhappy. Sheatsley and I were invited by a meeting of HIP staff physicians to tell them about the study. We did so and had a rather congenial evening, where the study was explained in detail. We published a condensed report in *Progress in Health Services,* which was widely publicized (Health Information Foundation, 1959). As usual, we had something for everybody—those who promoted group-practice plans, and those who provided fee-for-service plans. We submitted the report to the Harvard University Press, but it was turned down by a reviewer who appeared to be a group-practice prepayment proponent. We published it in our own research series (Anderson and Sheatsley, 1959). Our policy was that if regular publishers would not publish our reports, we would use our own research series. It sold well and as late as the 1970s and 1980s was in demand again, when group-practice plans were renamed health-maintenance organizations as the wave of the future.

In 1959, I was approached by the Massachusetts Blue Cross plan in Boston to do a study of the differences in cost per inpatient in Blue Cross plans compared with cost per inpatient in the private insurance plans. Blue Cross believed that its patients should have a lower cost than the private plans, for various reasons of efficiency, association with the hospitals, and mix of patients. Massachusetts had regulated that hospitals should charge all third-party payers the same rate. This was, in effect, a request that was suitable for a consulting agency, not a research agency. Seeing a chance to explore hospital utilization in an entire state, I said I would consider the kind of study Blue Cross wanted if I could gain entry to a statewide study of hospital utilization in the entire state. The foundation would finance the statewide study. This was agreed to by all parties concerned: the Massachusetts Hospital Association, the Massachusetts Medical Association, and the Blue Cross–Blue Shield plans. I therefore had powerful sanctioning agencies. At that time, Sol Levine was on the faculty of the Harvard School of Public Health, and he was engaged to do the "consulting" study and also worked with NORC and me on designing the statewide hospital-use study. The outcome of the cost-per-patient study was that actual costs, regardless of payer, were equal—to the disappointment of Blue Cross. Levine and I conducted a review in Boston with all principals and submitted the report.

The motivation for the statewide study was that the hospitals were increasingly being criticized for "overuse" of hospital care and were said to be largely responsible for the rising cost of health services—this, in 1959! Briefly, we made an elaborate survey of admissions, interviewing patients and their physicians not long after discharge from the hospitals. To oversimplify, the patients were queried about the sequence of events that led to hospitalization, and the attending physicians were queried about their perceptions, after the fact, of the relative need for admission to the hospital. The results were fascinating. For surgery, the attending physicians said that it would have been impossible for 74 percent of the patients to have had the surgery except in a hospital; for medical admissions, the proportion was 46 percent; for diagnostic admissions, it was 45 percent. The proportions for "extremely difficult except in a hospital" were 15 percent, 37 percent, and 32 percent, respectively. This left clearly discretionary decisions in 11, 17, and 23 percent of the cases, respectively. We suggested that these last percentages represented the very soft area of decision making, which could be eliminated without undue complaints from patients and physicians. Curiously and disappointingly, this study received very little attention as an empirical study of an important allegation: the overuse of hospitals. The condensed results were published in *Progress in Health Services* early in 1956 and in the research series after we moved to Chicago (Anderson and Sheatsley, 1967). I felt that this was one of the most sophisticated studies on this problem ever attempted. Maybe it was ahead of its time or beyond the possibility of the hospital administrators and medical staffs to implement.

Maturation of the Foundation

By 1959, the foundation had gained great respectability and visibility. At a meeting of the board of directors on May 10, 1957, we brought in researchers we had financed (such as Ethel Shanas, Nathan Sinai, and myself) to present the highlights of research in progress. The board appeared to be in a good mood. There was a discussion of the policy implications of the foundation's creating a film for television, to show the advances of and contributions to health of the medical sciences and the pharmaceutical industry. The conclusion was that it was too promotional and self-serving: "Objectivity and the middle course" must be maintained, so as not to jeopardize the foundation's tax-exempt status as an educational and research agency (Health Information Foundation, 1957).

George Smith, president of Johnson & Johnson, was the chairman of the board at that time. He reported that he and Bugbee, William Pollack, head of one of the labor unions, and Nelson Cruikshank, vice-president of the Social Security Committee of the AFL-CIO, had met for lunch (which the labor leaders paid for) to maintain contact with that particular interest group. Cruikshank told Smith that when the establishment of the Health Information Foundation was announced in 1950 Cruikshank believed that here was another research organization funded by a conservative business group to disseminate data and information unfavorable to government health insurance. Cruikshank had followed the research reports of the foundation and was pleased to observe that they were objective and straightforward. Smith was very pleased that the foundation was serving the purpose for which it was established (Health Information Foundation, 1957).

In April 1958, the *New England Journal of Medicine,* which could be characterized as moderately conservative in its political philosophy, published an editorial on the Health Information Foundation. To quote the editorial in part, "The Health Information Foundation, which has gone to work quietly in the establishment of facts relating to the distribution of medical care, was organized in 1950. Its founders were leaders in industry, especially those concerned with pharmaceutical, chemical and allied fields, and their belief was that progress in matters of health care can continue if citizens take the responsibility for the freedom to progress." The editorial went on to explain that the purpose of the foundation is to document research accomplishments of the current system of medical care, define areas in need of improvement, and publicize research results: "Already informational material is accumulating as a result of research studies made or initiated by the research director, Odin W. Anderson." Studies to date were listed (Editorial, 1958, p. 855).

In 1958, I was able to interest Duncan M. McIntyre, a professor of industrial relations at Cornell University, in doing a study of the issue of experience rating versus community rating, which had become a polemical battle between the nonprofit Blue plans and the for-profit private insurance companies. Originally, the Blue plans had charged the same premium for all employed groups enrolled in the community, in order to serve as a cross-subsidization agency, so that one group would not have a lower or higher premium than another group simply because of the accident of having more females or a more hazardous occupation, which resulted in higher risks actuarially. Private insurance companies competed by offering employers with low-risk employees a lower premium relative to the composition of the employees. This method broke the classic philosophy of the Blue plans as community plans. It was not known, however, what impact the differential premiums had on the cost sharing in the community. McIntyre made a definitive study of this issue and concluded that the impact of experience rating on market share was not as great as was assumed, and that the Blues had a range of flexibility that approximated a community rate. As a public policy, it was feared, widespread experience rating would make it costly for some employers to insure their groups, therefore limiting the overall coverage of the population with voluntary health insurance and making those left out dependent on public welfare (McIntyre, 1962).

Entrance into Cross-National Research

Bugbee and I had been discussing the possibility and advisability of my engaging in cross-national comparisons in the development and operation of health services delivery systems. Of most interest to Americans was the National Health Service (NHS) in Great Britain, which started in 1948. Next was Sweden, perceived as the "middle way" society. The idea was put to the board for me to go over on a short visit to scout the possibility of conducting a study. The board approved, and I flew over for three weeks in February 1958.

From my WHO fellowship trip, I had some good contacts in London who might give me some entrée and who might still remember me. I wrote to Professor Richard L. Titmuss of the London School of Economics, who in 1951 had been made the first professor of social administration in the world. He was essentially a philosopher of social policy and was a consultant to the Labor Party. I felt that he could be my starting point, and I could fan out from there to other informants, as suggested by him, and then fan out further to other informants suggested by the previous informants. I wrote to him about my reason for visiting and about how I wished to spend the short time I would be there. I quickly had a reply, and he invited me to dinner at his house in London on the day of my arrival. I met his wife, his daughter, and a graduate student in economics from Cambridge University who was working with Titmuss. The student was Brian Abel-Smith, who eventually became a well-known health economist and a consultant to the Labor Party. Both Titmuss and Abel-Smith were Fabian socialists, in the British tradition. The dinner was a most pleasant one, and I was complimented by their observation that my letter revealed more sophisticated knowledge of the NHS than other Americans who had come over. Titmuss was very helpful in suggesting knowledgeable informants and where to get official reports and literature. Titmuss seemed to be respected as a scholar and social philosopher across the Labor-Conservative spectrum. He also had an American graduate student, Frank Honigsbaum, who had been in London at the School of Economics for several years and who was very helpful. We spent many evenings together. Titmuss asked me if the foundation had some extra money to subsidize a book on the history of nursing in the United Kingdom, on which Abel-Smith was working. The sum requested was modest enough, and I could draw on the reserve fund I had for Ph.D. dissertations and other relatively small projects. In due course, that history of nursing became a classic.

I returned to New York with a vast quantity of reports and literature and notes from my numerous interviews. It was an intensive and rewarding three weeks. I immediately wrote a brief in-house descriptive analysis of the NHS for the staff and the board. I concluded that the NHS was successful within the British context.

The result of my interest in cross-national research was an annual trip in the fall to the United Kingdom and Scandinavia, particularly Sweden, until 1980, and sporadically thereafter. In 1960, I teamed up with Osler Peterson, then in the New York office of the Rockefeller Foundation and previously the Rockefeller Foundation representative for Europe, based in London. I had first met him in London on my WHO fellowship. We wished to explore together the possibility of cross-national comparative research in the United Kingdom and Sweden. I was after cross-national household surveys on the model developed with NORC. Peterson was more interested in small-area comparisons, and we split off after establishing research bases in Great Britain and Sweden.

In the fall of 1960, Peterson and I met with the director general of the Swedish board of health, Arthur Engel, a most congenial, tall, and robust person. We asked if there was interest in Sweden in comparative health services research. He said we had come just at the right time because a new professor of social medicine had just been appointed to the Faculty of Medicine at the University of Uppsala, forty miles north of Stockholm. He called this professor, Ragnar Berfenstam, immediately. Berfenstam was interested and met us the next day. We immediately started to plan joint projects. In Great Britain, Peterson began to plan joint projects with a social medicine physician from Manchester.

I tried to swing a three-country comparative nationwide household survey in the U.S., Great Britain, and Sweden. Berfenstam's department in Uppsala was interested immediately and got funds from the Swedish board of health. I got funds from the U.S. Public Health Service. My efforts in the U.K. to have the National Health Service bureaucracy cooperate in a comparative nationwide survey were most frustrating. I was even going to finance the survey from foundation funds and engage the Government Social Survey unit in London to conduct it. Titmuss was all for it because, as a socialist and a devout supporter of the National Health Service, he wanted to find out if access to health services had more or less equalized among income levels. The chief medical officer of the National Health Service, Sir George Godber, a pediatrician by specialty, was most interested in having the survey carried out. He said that I had made a generous offer. The survey could not, in all practicality, be carried out without the sanction of the top authorities of the National Health Service, as appeared to be the British custom. Also, the bureaucracy was more interested in operations research, to make the service more efficient and less costly, whereas it was the most frugal health service among the developed countries. The NHS apparently did not want a sociopolitical evaluation of whether it was attaining its egalitarian objectives. Sir George, a very warm and humane person, was most embarrassed when he was not able to convince the bureaucracy. Thus, we made a comparative study of the Swedish and the U.S. populations. In Great Britain, I continued, year after year, to assemble precollected official data and data from small-scale studies published by academics. A preliminary article on my work was requested by the *New England Journal of Medicine*, in two installments (Anderson, 1963).

What Now?

As I was opening up research in cross-national comparisons, the early and seemingly enthusiastic support of the foundation by the industry and the board began to weaken. There were two reasons for the new atmosphere. The founders of the foundation were not young men in 1950, when the foundation was chartered. By 1959, some had retired and had been replaced by younger men, who did not seem to have the patrician noblesse-oblige philosophy of the elders. A new generation of hard-nosed business types was taking over, and the mission of the foundation was not familiar to them. ("What good does it do directly to the pharmaceutical industry?") The other reason was the investigation of monopoly practices, possibly resulting in collusion on high prices for prescriptions, inaugurated by Senator Kefauver of Tennessee in 1959 (Kefauver, 1965). This shook the industry. Its profit margins were high, but the industry representatives said that the financial risks were also high. Some drugs paid off, others did not. Hearings on prescription drug prices were held by the Senate Subcommittee on Anti-Trust and Monopoly from December 1959 to 1962. The Kefauver-Harris legislation was introduced in October 1962, to regulate the safety of drugs, encourage generic drugs, and discourage costly advertising. At the few board meetings I attended, I felt that the members behaved almost as though they were in neutral territory, where they could engage in a public service away from the wear and tear of competition.

The change in the composition and leadership of the board and the Kefauver investigations spilled over to the value of continuing the foundation. Bugbee reported that there was a great deal of ambivalence. There was embarrassment about liquidating an agency that had so clearly established a reputation for objective social research, the results of which were generally sought by all parties. Bugbee and I had discussed the possibility of the industry's endowing the foundation in perpetuity with $10 million, which at 5 percent interest would yield the $500,000 we were accustomed to. Bugbee and I were not getting any younger. I was forty-five and he was fifty-five in 1959. We felt we needed more security. Nothing came of this idea. What the changed board did, however, was hire a well-known public relations firm, Cresap, McCormick and Paige, to evaluate our program and its future. The report, as far as Bugbee and I were concerned, turned out to be a typical public relations product, with little appreciation of the role of research, our reason for existence. We should consult interest groups about what we should do research on. We were doing that all the time, informally. We felt, however, that we knew the problems and issues in the field and their researchability better than anyone in the operational areas, without feeling too arrogant. That was our job. Bugbee and I discussed problems and issues all the time.

It became increasingly apparent, however, that our future was uncertain. We could not implement the vapid recommendations of the public relations agency, which did not understand our research mission. At the beginning of the Kefauver hearings, Bugbee and I were afraid we would be drawn in to tell the committee what a fine job the industry was doing in the public interest for $500,000 per year out of a gross income of $3 billion. Wisely, the board decided not to involve the foundation voluntarily in the hearings. It was not my role in relation to the industry.

Between 1959 and 1961, when it was rumored that the Health Information Foundation would be liquidated and Bugbee and I would throw ourselves on the market and I would seek an academic post, two universities approached us to move the foundation, its program, and its reserves (then about $1 million) to them. Coincidentally, Walter McNerney had resigned as director of the program in health services administration in the School of Business at the University of Michigan, to become executive director of the Blue Cross Association in Chicago. Ray Brown, superintendent of the University of Chicago Hospitals and Clinics and director of the program in hospital administration in the Graduate School of Business at the University of Chicago, resigned to become vice-president for maintenance at the university. Both universities began to talk to us about moving. Both universities were viable alternatives, but the University of Chicago's Graduate School of Business moved much more rapidly.

The industry and the board saw this development as an opportunity to unload the foundation gracefully. The rapid movement of Dean Allen Wallis of the Graduate School of Business at Chicago was most impressive. I was present at the board meeting where Wallis was selling the idea of having the foundation move to the University of Chicago. This was in 1961. What I remember most about Wallis's sales pitch was that the industry should realize that once a deal is made with the University of Chicago, the industry loses all control over the policy and operation of the foundation.

Another coincidence, in addition to the resignations of

McNerney and Brown, was that the Graduate School of Business at the University of Chicago was in the throes of reorganizing. The school had obtained a large grant from the Ford Foundation to reconstitute the school and its faculty. Among other things, the school was abolishing several industry-specific academic programs, such as meat packing and nursing, but had decided to retain the program in hospital administration, largely, I believe, because of the opportunity to get Bugbee as director and me as the research director of the foundation, plus around $1 million for our use. In three months or so, during the latter part of 1961, all decisions had been satisfactorily negotiated about space, rank, and salaries for Bugbee and me and for two core research staff members who would move with us. An important bonus for me was a courtesy appointment to the Department of Sociology, which gave me full academic privileges to teach and have graduate students in sociology as well as in the Graduate School of Business. Phillip Hauser of the Department of Sociology was helpful here. Not unexpectedly, given the culture of academia, particularly in prestige universities, rank and tenure were negotiated quite intensely. Bugbee, not having the usual academic credentials (such as a Ph.D. and scholarly publications), was made an untenured professor. After that decision, it was my turn, and Bugbee told the dean of the Graduate School of Business that if he did not satisfy me, the foundation would not move. I was then forty-seven years old, with academic continuity and many publications, but I was not able to swing a tenured professorship. The business faculty knew little about the health field, and the industry-specific program continued to be an anomaly in a business school oriented mainly to processes of management, no matter what was being managed. Bugbee said the best deal that could be made was to name me an associate professor and give me a five-year contract. I said, "Okay, but raise my salary to an average professor level." The dean said this might be difficult, but after a week of silence, my request was granted. The dean told me, however, that a tenured professorship, before the expiration of my five-year contract, was expected. Three months after I arrived, the dean resigned to become president of the University of Rochester. He was succeeded by George Shultz, later to be secretary of state. Within a year,

Shultz moved on this apparent promise, and I became a tenured professor in 1964. During this transition period, from about early 1960 to late 1961, the foundation maintained its research momentum. We had the money and the research ideas, which carried us over without a break during and after our move to the University of Chicago.

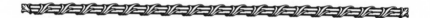

7

The University of Chicago, 1962–1980

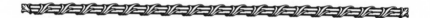

Moving the foundation from New York, as a freestanding national agency, to the University of Chicago Graduate School of Business, in an academic context, was an interesting experience in the evolution of the agency. Prior to my position as research director of the foundation, I had twelve years of experience with academic culture, although at a relatively low level in the hierarchy. Bugbee had no experience in that culture, having been mainly a health services and association administrator accustomed to hierarchical arrangements. At first, he found the academic culture mystifying. He said to me, "Professors do not return telephone calls." I think what he meant was that they do not return calls promptly. He was building relevant relationships within a structure, at which he was a past master. He quickly learned the characteristics of the academic culture. The University of Chicago facilitates a very freewheeling atmosphere for professors, particularly if they have financial resources to work with, as we did.

We had really strong support from the dean, George Shultz, and a small core of older and seasoned faculty, if not the enthusiastic support of the bulk of the faculty. Up to this time, the students concentrating in hospital administration had been regarded on the whole as not as good as the "regular" business students.

It was both strange and interesting to be plunked down onto this campus as a cohesive unit, which needed to work out relationships with a variety of faculties. The Health Information Foundation (later renamed the Center for Health Administration Studies, to conform to the university's usage of the term *center*) was an interdisciplinary research center and thus was intended to attract Ph.D. students and faculty researchers who were interested in conducting health-related research projects. Building relationships took time. Professors, very much so at the University of Chicago, create baronies; their graduate students are the front-line troops. We attracted attention by our continuing research and continuing connections with NORC. Gradually, we attracted Ph.D. students to use the Center for Health Administration Studies (CHAS) as a research base, and we also provided some seed money. Over the subsequent years, I was invited to participate on Ph.D. committees all over the university, for dissertations that had some health services relevance. We became the medical sociology component of the Department of Sociology.

I was asked to be on the board that created the Hyde Park–Kenwood Community Health Center, a primary-care clinic that later became affiliated with an HMO. It took five years of meetings at the local YMCA to get off the ground. It was a great learning process for community board members who had little knowledge of the complexities of medical administration. Patience was needed. We had a dazzling chairman, Lawrence Bloom, who later became an alderman on the Chicago City Council.

In research, we continued to move into nationwide household surveys and cross-national ventures. Projects started in New York—such as the second nationwide household survey of use and expenditures by my associates and me, the nationwide household survey of the elderly by Shanas, the attitude study by Feldman, and the Massachusetts hospital-use study by Sheatsley and me—were published after we moved to Chicago and enabled us to show a continuing momentum. The assemblage of vital statistical trends started by Monroe Lerner and me in New York was organized into a book, with Lerner as senior author (Lerner, 1963). It was published by the University of Chicago Press. (Lerner joined the research staff of the Blue Cross Association in Chicago.)

We tried to continue the ten annual issues of *Progress in Health Services* at the Chicago site. We tried to rotate bulletins among the staff and also hired an editor, Kong Kyun Ro, to write bulletins and coordinate them with staff members. We found, however, that the discipline for a monthly bulletin of the quality we wanted was really not practical in an academic setting. We found that the deadlines harassed the staff, taking them away from ongoing research projects, and we gave the publication up.

In the 1960s and into the 1970s, it was quite easy to get grants for health services research. It will be recalled that the surveys in 1953 and 1958 were financed by the pharmaceutical industry, through the Health Information Foundation. After we moved to the University of Chicago, a third nationwide household survey was indicated, given the continuing dynamism of the health services field. Another survey was floated in 1963, financed by the Health Information Foundation and by a grant from the U.S Public Health Service. This grant of $400,000 included plans to establish working relationships with Swedish and British colleagues.

Funds were offered by the Ford Foundation, amounting to $75,000 for general research seed money and the continuation of *Progress in Health Services.* The grant was also used as seed money for Ph.D. dissertations, both internally and externally. The money was not even requested from the Ford Foundation. One of its representatives came around, looked at our activities, and offered the $75,000. We also got grants from the Kellogg Foundation for the Program in Hospital Administration, to cover teaching costs. This foundation was helping health services administration programs in universities in various parts of the country to get started—or, in our case, to improve.

The Health Information Foundation was still chartered in Illinois as an agency through which the pharmaceutical industry might still continue to contribute money. In fact, after we moved to Chicago, we were given, over a three-year period, around $350,000, after which the flow stopped. The Health Information Foundation went out of existence as a legal entity in 1971. We also continued to regard the $1 million reserve we had brought with us from New York as an endowment, spending little of the capital and using the interest for various purposes. One of them was the funding of my annual trips to Europe, to build and maintain a network of contacts, follow the trends in their respective health services, and keep on gathering reports and data. I simply wrote a memorandum to the comptroller's office every year, requesting an advance for each trip.

We continued the research series we had started in New York. The Graduate School of Business thus empowered us to publish research reports by the staff rapidly, without the slowness of reviews of publishing houses and professional journals. We were our own jurors. Reports that were not particularly urgent were published in the usual outlets. Once, a site visit of peers sent out by the National Center for Health Services Research was criticized for not having the research reports reviewed by peers. I replied that researchers who are engaged in policy-oriented research are criticized by the users of such research for taking so long to disseminate results that by the time they are available, the policy issue has been resolved without research. Further, and somewhat arrogantly, I said that our staff was sufficiently sophisticated and competent to stand behind the quality of the research, without submitting our reports to peer review. My experience with peer review of our work in New York and later in Chicago was that health services research was so interdisciplinary that reviewers from a particular discipline were not able to see the report as a whole and its policy implications.

On the whole, we had good relationships with the governmental funding agencies important to our work—for example, the Bureau of Health Services Research (up to 1965), which became part of the National Center for Health Services Research. We were regarded as having a good record in choice of research problems, production, and scheduling.

Research Funding Stabilized

In 1965, we were fortunate in applying for and getting a seven-year programmatic grant from the bureau (carrying over to the National Center for Health Services Research later). The grant amounted to about $1.16 million for program support and development to help maintain the center, with no particular research projects being required. This gave us stability to apply for project grants from one source or another. Our site was visited in 1967 for a review of progress, and the grant was continued for the entire seven years.

By the time I took on the third nationwide household survey, in 1963, I was quite punch-drunk from floating and writing up such surveys, but the health field found them useful. Economists became interested in household data, even though these data did not seem as "hard" to them as economic data reported by business and government. We produced the only consumer data to be broken down by both family and individual units. Fortunately, I was largely relieved of the details of supervising the 1963 survey by hiring a graduate student in sociology from Purdue University, Ronald Andersen, who was then twenty-four years old and looking for a dissertation topic. I was hoping that Andersen would turn out to be competent and willing to take over the entire project and be the senior author, although I did not tell him so at the time. After working with Andersen for six months and observing how he related to NORC, I asked him if he would like to take on the senior responsibility for the survey. He moved right into it and built on the previous surveys. For example, a list of symptoms and whether or not a physician had been seen for them was added (Andersen and Anderson, 1967). Andersen also used the data for his Ph.D. dissertation, devising a behavioral model of families' use of health services (Andersen, 1968). This model has been referred to and applied by many other sociologists, in one of the usually rare instances when a dissertation makes a major contribution to a field and is published with few revisions.

The move to the University of Chicago gave me a firmer base for long-term projects. One was to write a sociopolitical history of the development of the American health services. The other was to write a book on cross-national comparisons of selected health services delivery systems in developed liberal-democratic countries, beginning with the U.K. and Sweden, where I had already made a start in the fall of 1958. Concurrently with my venture into cross-national research, in 1962 I started to give a course on the development of the American health services, researching madly as I went along, only a month or so ahead of my lectures. That book was published in 1968 (Anderson, 1968b).

When I hired Andersen, I extended the scope of this survey to include a parallel survey of the Swedish population, to see if we could determine what influence differences in the organizational structures of the delivery systems might have on utilization patterns. We collaborated with Bjorn Smedby in the Department of Social Medicine at the University of Uppsala. Using the same survey instrument in two or more languages is a tricky business when the information to be gathered from informants in different languages deals with subjective and emotional elements, such as perceptions of illness and health. In due course, we published the first cross-national comparisons of the operation of health services delivery systems in two countries, the United States and Sweden (Andersen, Smedby, and Anderson, 1970). An interesting finding, contrary to our hypothesis, was that the number of symptoms reported had a similar relationship to utilization in the two countries, indicating similarity in perception of symptoms.

Papers and Studies Commissioned by Interested Agencies

In 1966, the American Institute of Planners (AIP) sponsored a futuristic project to predict what would and should happen in fourteen areas of public policy during the fifty years from 1967 to 2017. These areas covered a gamut of concerns, such as education, housing, urban structure, manpower, transportation, natural resources, the arts, and health. People regarded as experts in these areas were invited to write futuristic papers. I was invited to write the paper on the health field. William R. Ewald, Jr., was the project administrator, who sent out the invitations late in 1966. I readily accepted, feeling very honored. The general content desired by the AIP was as follows:

> This paper was commissioned to weigh our choices for the good life, to examine the costs and rewards of physical and mental health for all people of all ages. At which point is man's ability to adapt to his man-made environment too costly in human health terms? Can we afford good health for all? Which priority should there be for research? What are the great innovations to be made? What institutional changes will be required? Does health for all mean bureaucracy for all? Is that a price we *have* to pay? Are the aged to exist

or live, and how? How can public health practices catch up to the foreseeable needs? What sort of deliberate genetic control do we want or need?

Obviously, the foregoing gave wide scope to the writer, but this would be tempered and challenged by the AIP's appointment of a committee of ten leading authorities in public health, medical care, health services, organization, and finance, who would read the draft and submit critiques. One could then revise the paper as one saw fit and resubmit it to the members of the committee who had made rejoinders. The members of the committee—an impressive group, active people with faith in their opinions, for an academic researcher to take on—were then privileged to eliminate or revise their rejoinders. The remarks of those who still felt at odds with the writer would be included in footnotes or appendixes. In my case, publication was guaranteed, no matter how I responded to the critiques.

I took the global objectives implicit in the AIP's statement as the rhetoric of optimism, not realizing that the sponsors seemed to take them seriously. I assumed that they wanted a freewheeling, more or less personal treatment. When my writing outline was delivered, two of the committee members were distressed. They did not like my acceptance of the incremental political bargaining and negotiating inherent in the American political process (indeed, the same style, with variations, characteristic of all liberal democracies). They did recognize that this style was a political reality, but they had hoped for a statement of rational, technocratic change. The concept of planning was then becoming popular, but I had little faith in planning as conceived by technocrats. In fact, I was fearful of technocrats. I believe they were familiar with my household surveys of expenditures and utilization patterns—which planners, of course, like very much. I believe they thought that I did not understand my task. I had not yet started to write on health services policy and the liberal-democratic political process in this country and abroad. Retrospectively, I feel that my AIP essay did not become a neat statistical document of need, demand, and costs, as had been expected; no one had written this way in health policy before.

The theory of pluralistic democracy aside, I also visualized a generously proportioned health services financing and delivery system. The population was aging, more effective medical technology was appearing, and prevention was being encouraged, including the exhortation to "see your doctor" early. All of these trends would impinge heavily on the cost trends. Recall that this was in 1967, in the euphoria of President Johnson's war on poverty and illness. By this time, however, the first glimmers of concern with the rising cost of health services were appearing within public policy debates. The federal and state governments were then responsible for Medicare and Medicaid, enacted in 1965, and the usual underestimation of eventual costs was distressing government. Medicare was being financed by a payroll tax on employers and employees, Medicaid from general revenues of the federal and state governments.

Drawing on a heuristic model in my head, as a gestalt of ponderables and imponderables, and not an econometric model, throwing in selected variables over time, I predicted that the percentage of gross national product (GNP) allocated to the health services would rise from the 6 percent of 1965 to 9 percent in 1980 and stabilize until 2017. I wrote that this growth was necessary if we were to have loosely enough structured and financed health services to provide a relatively reasonable amount and quality of care, be relatively convenient of access, and have no unduly long waiting lists. The members of the committee who responded agreed that we should have a generously proportioned health service, but that it need not cost as much as I had predicted; I had paid little attention to the need to reorganize the pluralistic structure of the current delivery system, but by so doing, we could have a generously proportioned health service at a lower cost.

It is true that in 1967 I had not anticipated the rapid growth of HMOs, nor had anyone else. Notwithstanding this turn of events, I again, as with planning, have never intuitively had much faith in the capacity of organizational structures to ensure meaningful cost containment. The forces pressing on the health services infrastructure were too powerful to be contained by structure. Costs can be contained only by tight budgets, rationing, and waiting lists.

This view was, of course, too pessimistic for my usually optimistic colleagues on the committee, who had faith in structure. Now, as is known, it turns out that I underestimated the increase in the percentage of GNP allocated to health services. It now stands at almost 12 percent. What I was not wrong on, however, was that subsequent developments of HMOs in structure and competition have not been spectacular successes in containing costs, either.

In any case, the surgeon general of the U.S. Public Health Service invited me and the members of the committee, with a few members of the Public Health Service staff, for a day of discussion of my essay in Washington, on May 4, 1967. This was a strenuous but rewarding experience, in a quite congenial and collegial atmosphere. Throughout there were spirited exchanges between me and the chairman of the committee and the consultant and program chairman for AIP. My essay was published in the AIP publication and in our own research series at the Center for Health Administration Studies, University of Chicago (see Ewald, 1968; Anderson, 1968a).

We were also requested by the American College of Hospital Administrators (ACHA), now the American College of Health Care Executives (ACHCE), to do a consulting project. In 1970, Richard Stull, the president of ACHA, conferred with me about helping ACHA examine the concept of some form of universal governmental health insurance, which at that time was under constant consideration by Congress and was regarded as inevitable and imminent. A very prestigious board of eleven members was appointed, all hospital administrators. There were several bills proposed, but none reached the floor of Congress for debate. In any case, ACHA was apprehensive of its implications, if enacted, for hospital administrators throughout the country, who would have the major problem of implementing whatever might be enacted. ACHA was not intending to oppose the enactment of a universal health insurance plan, if that emerged as part of the American political process and as the apparent will of the people. What ACHA's members feared was the enactment of a bill that would be difficult to administer; thus, they would be blamed if the bill did not meet expectations. Stull wanted a systematic statement of the public policy issues and a synthesis of the views of scores of administrators on what the legislation should entail, so as to make it as operable as possible. This was a very statesmanlike and professional approach, which I helped ACHA to formulate.

The consulting grant was generous and enabled me to gather a good staff of four for a twelve-month project. The associate director, Sheldon Bergman, interviewed hospital executives all over the country and in Canada (which had had a nationwide hospital insurance plan since 1958). He personally interviewed 128 administrators, including the members of the Study Commission in forty-four states and five Canadian provinces. A professional writer, Harry Dreiser, the publicity writer for the dean of the Graduate School of Business, and I synthesized the interview reports. Other staff members were two graduate students in political science and a graduate of the Program in Hospital Administration.

The eleven members of the Study Commission were brought in one by one to my office in the Center for Health Administration Studies and vigorously interviewed for a couple of hours each about their concepts of administration, health insurance, and problems of implementation as hospital administrators. I recall that they enjoyed this "interrogation" immensely. They said they rarely had a chance in their hectic lives to be forced to organize their thoughts and raise their level of consciousness. The report submitted to the Study Commission was used as an empirical and conceptual basis for recommendations to Congress and policymakers on how a universal health insurance bill should be drafted, so that it could be managed well. This work on national health insurance and its implications for the management of hospitals proceeded very smoothly at every stage and was well received. A contrasting experience was the project that Joel May and I took on for the Blue Cross–Blue Shield Associations.

Late in 1960, the Blue Cross and Blue Shield Associations, the national federations of the Blue plans, approached me about the possibility of studying the operation of the Federal Employees Health Benefits Program (FEHBP) as a potential model that could be used in the event of the enactment of some kind of national health insurance. The FEHBP had been in operation since 1960, when Congress, like any other employer, established the program for federal civil servants. The program was ardently supported by the existing health insurance agencies, since there was a potential market for eight million members, including dependents.

Briefly, the federal employees were given a choice among the

Blue Cross and Blue Shield plans, private insurance, and group-practice prepayment. Each of these insurers placed a bid with the Civil Service Commission (CSC), which was the government's administrative agency. The CSC specified standards of range of benefits, which included low-cost and higher-cost options. The premiums for the low-cost options were to be paid in full by the government. For higher-cost options with richer benefits, the federal employees would pay out-of-pocket expenses. The CSC sent quite elaborate information brochures to all federal employees, so that they could choose their particular plans with facts in hand.

By 1970, there were almost ten years of experience with the FEHBP, which was well regarded by all interested parties. Blue Cross–Blue Shield had a fair share of this business, hence its interest in a study of performance in general and comparative performance of the various choices. No overall evaluation had been done before.

With the essential interest and cooperation of Joel May, who was then associate director of the Center for Health Administration Studies and a capable researcher and statistician, I agreed to undertake the study commissioned by the associations through the Health Services Foundation. Almost all the data, plan by plan, were owned by the CSC for each year since 1960, covering enrollment, costs, and utilization. The time pressure was intense. This endeavor was in the form of a contract, rather than a grant. The funds were quite adequate for the purpose. The understanding was that, as an independent university research agency, we would produce a study that, as far as empirically possible, would show the performance levels of the various plans and speculate about using the FEHBP model for universal health insurance or for the information of the big buyers of services (large industries).

The first draft of the study was delivered to the appropriate representatives of the Blue Cross–Blue Shield Associations early in 1971, on time. Joel May and I met with a committee of representatives, who suggested we change this or that—nothing of dire significance, as I recall. The people we met with were not top officials but public relations–oriented, lower personnel, who seemed to be nervous about straightforward candor, for which I had a reputation and, presumably, the reason why I was approached to do the study. One specific observation on their part concerned the use of the word *trepidation,* which we used in connection with the differences in cost of administration relative to income to compare costs of administration among the various plans. They did not want us to express any uncertainty or equivocation about the validity of our data, some of which, as in all studies, needed to be qualified. Thus, we took out *trepidation* and used a milder word. As we left the meeting, May was furious and wanted to cancel the contract and return the money. I was twenty-five years his senior, and he had been one of my students, so I told him to "hang in there" and see if we could not iron out differences in perception. The understanding was that we would have the right to publish, even if the study, for some reason or another, was not acceptable to the associations. The associations had sent the draft of the study to executives in local state plans. One had expected a "lively, vibrant history." Another wrote that the report was not up to my usual standards. There was little, empirically, to be "vibrant" about, because the study was a straightforward statistical report with guarded interpretations, given the relative paucity of and the nature of the data, which had not been gathered for research purposes. I am sure I was approached because I was regarded as being "neutral on their side." The statistical information did not reveal startling differences among the various plans—except, as expected, there was appreciably lower use of hospital days in the group-practice plans, compared with the other plans, an important exception, for the so-called independent, fee-for-service medical plans also had relatively low use of hospitals (Anderson and May, 1971).

The second draft was not acceptable, either. A cordial letter from a vice-president of the Blue Cross Association, whom I knew well, stated: "The best way for me to express the group consensus, Odin, seems just to say that 'it didn't come off.' I suppose this is always a problem between a group that has an idea of something it would like to see written, and the end product. But as we review the second effort, it is our joint conclusion that the report doesn't say what we hoped it might say, and perhaps it can't be done, but in any case we don't feel that another rewrite of this approach would accomplish it." Under the circumstances, it was not surprising that the associations would not pay the costs of publication, although in no sense whatsoever were we told not to publish. They were willing, moreover, to be acknowledged as the source of funds.

When our report was published by the Center for Health Administration Studies, late in 1971, there was a reaction. In December 1971, the Group Health Association of America issued a special supplement of its news publication. The medical consultant to GHAA, W. Palmer Dearing, M.D., whom I knew well, was disturbed by the relatively high administrative cost attributed to the group-practice prepayment plans, with the exception of the independent plans, and by the revelation, which was new information, that the independent plans were coming close to the low-hospital-use patterns of the group-practice plans. GHAA had touted both its comparatively low administrative costs and its hospital use as selling points. As usual, the attack was methodological and statistical. There were methodological niceties that, if redefined or manipulated, would have made minor changes, but not enough to modify the substance of our results for policy implications. May and I wrote a rejoinder, which was printed in an issue of the GHAA news publication along with a rebuttal from Dearing, which repeated the criticism of the statistical treatment. In a letter of January 3, 1972, I wrote: "I find the tenor of the critique difficult to understand, in view of the generally favorable comparisons the group-practice plans show. During the 1950s, I was attacked by the AMA in a special article by Frank Dickinson. The GHAA attack now seems to balance the polar attitudes."

I learned later that the GHAA, at the moment of publication of my report, was preparing for a new enrollment period. What this reveals is the charged atmosphere of the time, as the various plans competed vigorously for the federal employees' market. Any data throwing the slightest doubt on the group-practice plans' performance (even though these still compared favorably with their competitors) were feared. Not long after, I saw Dearing at a meeting. He was very friendly, as if nothing had taken place. He had tried to erode my credibility. I had always been friendly with GHAA members and had attended their annual meetings frequently. What I learned was that the attack was not personal; it was simply an interest group's protection of its interests.

GHAA and its group-practice members had always assumed

a "holier than thou" attitude toward plans that, presumably, were not as devoted to the public interest as the group plans were. I should have anticipated the consequences of these findings, but I thought the data were such that no one plan needed to feel threatened. In any case, absolutely nothing more came of this episode. I interacted with group-practice prepayment people as if this unpleasant episode had not taken place at all.

In 1970, I was approached by Walter J. McNerney, then president of the Blue Cross Association, about writing a book on the history of the Blue Cross development. Actually, he asked me if I knew of a professional historian who might want to write one. I said I did not know of such a historian, but I knew of an amateur historian who would like to write one—namely, me. He seemed pleased with my offer and suggested that I prepare a proposal, a schedule, and a budget. He said his objective was to have a book that would preserve the institutional memory of the Blue Cross movement for current and future Blue Cross leaders. I was quite familiar with early and contemporary Blue Cross leaders and with the development of Blue Cross plans when I was with Sinai at the University of Michigan.

He expected a straightforward and objective history of the movement, granting me all academic freedom. He had once been in an academic post himself. He set one condition—which I had not yet thought of, because of travel expenses—that I should hurry and personally interview all starters of Blue Cross plans wherever they might be; most of them were already retired. This was a welcome request.

I quickly submitted my proposal, to which he responded immediately. He said that the proposal was good, but I had not asked for enough money. He wanted to make sure that I would not have an alibi for not doing a thorough job for lack of funds (a common complaint of researchers), particularly with respect to travel funds for interviews. My first budget was $25,000; my second was $33,000. McNerney submitted my proposal to the association, and it was approved. I engaged two graduate research assistants. My travel costs exceeded all the other costs. I interviewed over thirty Blue Cross starters, from New York to California and from Minnesota to Louisiana. Many times when I had a day off, I flew to my informant and back the same day. It was fun because my informants were a happy lot. They felt that they had performed a public service by starting nonprofit Blue Cross hospital plans. All interviews were taped, and they now repose in the archives of the Blue Cross–Blue Shield Association (the two associations eventually merged).

It took some time to find a publisher, even with a subsidy from the project. Beacon Press was interested until its reviewer pointed out that Yale University Press had published a book by Sylvia Law that was critical of the Blue Cross plans for not really serving the public interest (Law, 1974). My book was more sympathetic and not critical enough. Beacon Press rejected my manuscript like a hot potato. Eventually, Ballinger accepted the manuscript (Anderson, 1975).

The Chicago Emergency Medical Care Study

In 1968, CHAS became involved in a research-consultancy capacity with the medical emergency services of the Chicago metropolitan area. Both nationwide and in the Chicago area, there had been a great increase in the number of visits to emergency rooms of general hospitals. Individual hospitals were reporting substantial increases in visits to emergency rooms and in the proportion of patients with nonacute conditions. The emergency rooms were largely becoming the primary-care facilities for an increasing number of low-income patients. Early in 1968, several incidents took place in Chicago that led various agencies and individuals to issue public statements to redefine the responsibility of hospitals regarding emergency service. The news media reported several incidents of mismanagement.

The interested and affected parties began to mobilize. Recommendations had been introduced in the Chicago City Council to designate and establish trauma centers (a new category of emergency care) for severely traumatized accident victims, particularly of automobile accidents. Changes in the state law were being sought by the Illinois Hospital Licensing Board, which would have the effect of conditionally abolishing the requirement that all hospitals provide emergency medical service. Further, hospital administrators complained that the low collection rate from patients, privately or from public sources, was resulting in financial losses in their emergency departments. The policy was being formulated to create a regional network of trauma centers in designated hospitals in the Chicago metropolitan area.

In response, the Chicago Hospital Council (the federation of hospitals in the Chicago area) convened a conference on May 15, 1968, jointly sponsored by the Chicago Board of Health. Agencies represented at this conference included the Chicago Committee on Trauma of the American College of Surgeons, the Chicago Medical Society, Cook County Hospital, the Hospital Licensing Board of the State of Illinois, the Hospital Planning Council for Metropolitan Chicago, the Illinois Regional Medical Program, the Institute of Medicine of Chicago, and the Welfare Council of Metropolitan Chicago. It is clear that emergency services had become a public issue in the area. A wide range of topics was discussed, such as interhospital communication, public and private ambulance systems, interhospital transfers, hospital emergency departments, and reimbursement. Of interest is that the only consensus to emerge from the conference was that any changes and plans suggested must be based on facts, rather than on intuition.

The conferees requested that the Chicago Hospital Council form a steering committee, that a study proposal be formulated, that staff for the study be recruited, and that financing for the study be sought. The steering committee was formed by the Chicago Hospital Council in June 1968, representing a wide range of public and private agencies involved with emergency medical services in Chicago. Financing was obtained from the Illinois Regional Medical Program, the Chicago Medical Society, the Community Trust of Chicago, and member hospitals of the Chicago Hospital Council. The steering committee requested that CHAS prepare a study proposal.

This request was, of course, a great compliment. We were recognized by the health services establishment as a university research unit oriented toward policy research and were regarded as neutral. We therefore had immediate sponsorship by influential agencies and entry to their records and interview sources of data. Further, they provided quite ample research funds, in the range of $200,000 or so.

Undoubtedly, the main personal attraction to the sponsors was the presence of George Bugbee, director of CHAS and of the Program in Hospital Administration. Bugbee, as noted earlier, had countless influential contacts among administrators, hospital associations, and medical associations. He and I became joint principal investigators, and we hired a project director, Geoffrey Gibson, a Ph.D. in sociology from Ohio State University. Gibson was a fortunate find because he took charge of the study methodology and final report fast and furiously.

This study was, in sociological jargon, *action research*. We were in periodic contact with the steering committee of the Chicago Hospital Council. On occasion, as the study progressed, we had meetings with representatives of the agencies just mentioned. When the report was completed, we staged a grand review of the findings and the forty-eight recommendations for improving the emergency medical services of the Chicago metropolitan area. From this report emerged the concept of regional hospital trauma centers and its implementation in the 1960s.

In addition to Bugbee, Gibson, and me, we assembled a research and supporting staff of twenty-four. All sources of data were exploited: exhaustive literature review; comparative case materials from American cities and from Australia to Moscow; collection of hospital data forms; questionnaires to hospitals; on-site hospital surveys; logbook abstracts from emergency departments; surveys of private and public ambulances; abstracts of fire department and police department ambulance runs; interviews of patients in emergency departments; and cost studies. Our interviewers were permitted to ride ambulances on their runs. All of them reported exciting experiences. Gibson himself was an "urban animal," a very streetwise social researcher.

The final report was a mine of information on the systemic characteristics of medical emergency service in the Chicago metropolitan area. No such intensive survey had ever been done of a metropolitan area before, nor has there been one since. It was a town-and-gown cooperative effort. The report did not develop a theoretical systems framework on how the various parts were interrelated, but it did assemble a well-organized reservoir of data on the various elements of the medical emergency system in the area.

To this extent, the many actors could see themselves in a larger framework than before (Gibson, Bugbee, and Anderson, 1971).

Change in Directorship

In 1970, George Bugbee retired from the Graduate School of Business and as director of the Center for Health Administration Studies and the Program in Hospital Administration. His retirement broke the continuity of the custom by which the director of the Program in Hospital Administration was a statesman-administrator, serving as a role model for students who would become hospital and medical care administrators.

For a time, in contemplating Bugbee's retirement, we were thinking of ways to get closer to the medical school and to the hospitals and clinics of the University of Chicago with our seating in the Graduate School of Business. An academic physician interested in health services administration and research was sought. We found Robert Daniels, a professor of psychiatry working mainly in social and community psychiatry. Joel May was engaged as associate director of the program. I retained my position as associate director of the center and research director. I had no interest in being director of the center. It would pull me away from my research time. The dean of the Graduate School of Business agreed with my view. Daniels, however, was director of the center only a year or so. He became dean of the School of Medicine at the University of Cincinnati.

The position of director of the center was thrown open again. The dean of the school told me that I was not a candidate (nor did I wish to be), because he feared that the position would jeopardize my research production. I said, however, I would consider being the director if no suitable and willing candidate could be found, in order to give the center continuity. The dean himself assumed the title of acting director during the interim. We did have research and program activities going on, to keep us occupied, without any major decisions for a short interim, at least. Nine months passed in this limbo. One late afternoon, in March 1972, he called me at my home and said I had been appointed director of the center. May became director of the program and associate director of the center. He really ran the day-to-day activities and staff of the center and relieved me of many details. In 1978, he accepted a position with the New Jersey Hospital Association and resigned.

I replaced May with Richard Foster, a Ph.D. in the Graduate School of Business and the program, who had been working with May. Foster became an associate director of the program, and I became director. Thus, I assumed the same responsibilities as Bugbee had before his retirement. The center maintained something of an even keel, but the Bugbee type of leadership was missed, although this type was regarded as passé in a very academically oriented research institution. I presumably fit the academic model.

The period from 1970 to 1980 was one when several projects were completed and published, reflecting the buildup from the previous decade. An important project, building on the previous household surveys of 1953, 1958, and 1963, was the final household survey, floated in 1970, with funding that had been obtained from the National Center for Health Services Research in 1969, while Bugbee was still at his post. This survey was conducted by Andersen and became his second household survey, with some refinements. The final product from this survey was a synthesis of all the previous surveys, enabling a graphic picture of trends in the American health services over a twenty-year period. This survey became the last one of this type conducted by the Center for Health Administration Studies (Andersen, Lion, and Anderson, 1976).

By this time, the U.S. Center for Health Statistics was conducting periodic surveys in use, expenditures, and morbidity. A federal governmental agency was thus beginning to assume the legitimate function of providing statistics periodically for general consumption. This type of survey was no longer politically controversial. The Health Information Foundation and the Center for Health Administration Studies had shown the value of these surveys for policy formulation.

Changing Policies of Funding Agencies

By the end of the 1960s and into the 1970s, it was beginning to become more difficult to obtain research funds for health services research or, for that matter, other fields. Funding agencies, both private and public, were being staffed by people who had research competence and who began to negotiate with academically based researchers about choice of research problems, scope of research, and even methodology. Greater specifications were being requested, bordering on a contract between the funding agency staff and the academic researchers seeking funds. We in academic positions began to feel pressured—probably overreacting, considering our previous freewheeling relations, as represented by programmatic grants like the seven-year one CHAS obtained in 1965. Funding agencies were trying to ensure that they got what they paid for, of the scope agreed to, delivered on time.

The new attitude became apparent when we were negotiating with the National Center for Health Services Research (NCHSR) for the funding of the 1970 survey. Over the years, we had gotten to know the staff well as research colleagues with common interests. The survey research methodology in household surveys of use, expenditures, and morbidity had attained a high degree of standardization, which could be stipulated in a research contract. In this instance, the negotiations pushed the boundaries of specificity far beyond those we had been accustomed to.

I flew to Washington to put the final touches to the contract for the 1970 survey (which would actually be conducted at the end of 1970, for a twelve-month retrospective collection of data from informants). As I was reviewing the fine print and specifications of the contract with a whole long table full of federal agency representatives, I noted that there was a specification that the funding agency had the right to approve the final draft of the report from the survey, implying that a draft regarded as unsatisfactory could be refused publication. I asked, "What is this about?" There was a somewhat embarrassed response that the specification was only a technicality, which among colleagues would not matter. I said that we were colleagues, but that there was such a high turnover in staff that they might not be my colleagues by the time this survey was completed. It was explained that this contract specification was a spillover, so to speak, of all contracts with the federal government, from fighter planes to highway construction to research. These were hardware quality controls, to ensure that the contractor was delivering what was specified.

I said I would not approve this contract (for several hundred thousand dollars) if this specification remained in. I had to have the right to publish, no matter what, given my position as an academic. I was asked if the University of Chicago contract office would not accept the contract as written. I said that *I* did not accept the contract, whether the University of Chicago accepted it or not (knowing the university would not, according to its policy). We agreed to hold the contract in abeyance until I got back to Chicago to consult with the university contract office. Back at the University of Chicago, I called the chief of the contract office, told him what had happened in Washington, and sought his counsel. He said, "Odin, if that contract comes to my desk without that unwanted specification having been removed, I will reject the contract." I said, "Good. Where do we go from here?" He said, "Do you want to take it from here, or shall I deal directly with Washington?" I said, "You do." He did, and that specification was removed.

In the meantime, the seven-year programmatic grant starting in 1965 was to expire in 1972. Our site had been visited by the National Center for Health Services Research and Development in 1967. Several staff members, plus faculty in other parts of the Graduate School of Business, had conducted research, financed by the programmatic grant, on a range of problems. Before the expiration date, we applied for another programmatic grant. A quite elaborate site visit from the National Center for Health Services Research and Development was assembled at the University of Chicago on July 12, 1972. We applied for a five-year grant totaling about $1,350 million, including indirect costs of $211,000. With little haggling, the programmatic grant was renewed for five years, until 1978, for the amount requested. (Recall that the programmatic grant was to maintain continuity of the center and staff, who in addition to small grants from the programmatic grant, could generate research projects funded from other sources as well. One such grant, secured in 1973 from the Social Rehabilitation Service and the Social Security Administration of the federal government, was to study the effect of hospital organization on hospital efficiency and quality of medical care by three researchers, two at the University of Chicago's Graduate School of Business and one an alumnus of the center, then at Harvard University. The grant was for $115,000.)

A research proposal that was not approved during this period was a repeat of the emergency medical care study of the Chicago metropolitan area, with additional analyses, such as referral patterns of physicians to hospital emergency departments and the extent of implementation of the many recommendations leading to the establishment of regional trauma centers. Apparently, the project was not approved because of criticisms of this methodology. The original emergency study was regarded as too descriptive, and our proposal was criticized as not sufficiently laying out in great methodological detail how we would design the overall project and subprojects.

It is of interest to note that this was the first time a proposal of ours had been turned down for methodological reasons (although there may have been other reasons not mentioned). Up to this time, the Center for Health Administration Studies had been trusted to produce research, on the basis of the record of the staff and myself— to design and execute a project, with little doubt about our methodology as long as we promised the delivery of a final product that would be a practical contribution to the field. It seemed that funder-researcher relationships were changing toward a contract specification including the methodology-research relationship.

My impression was that both public and philanthropic funding sources were becoming more directly mission-oriented and wished to engage university-based research centers somewhat as extensions of their own missions, since they usually did not have research staffs themselves. I also had the impression that, along with mission-oriented objectives, the funding agencies had experienced some indifference on the part of university-based researchers to meet production deadlines.

Early in 1975, the NCHSR announced a new policy for the promotion of health services research. Apparently, instead of continuing the type of programmatic grant that we had been operating on since 1965, the NCHSR was floating a new arrangement, by which it would establish research centers in a number of universities for an indefinite period by having universities compete for a center. The concept was to have some kind of working relationship between the NCHSR and the recipient university. Also stipulated was that such a research center should establish working relationships with delivery systems, to facilitate the choice of research ideas and feed research results directly into operating delivery systems. NCHSR was to formulate guidelines for applicants, to help them write up formal applications. It was apparent that NCHSR was trying to have some influence over the relatively free choice of research problems we enjoyed in our programmatic grants, as well as over programs in other universities that NCHSR was funding. It seemed to us that we had developed a type of a model that, if adapted to the specifications and guidelines that might be proposed by NCHSR, would have a good chance of being awarded a programmatic grant.

The dean of the Graduate School of Business, Richard Rossett, was somewhat wary of the approach taken by NCHSR as interfering with research prerogatives in the Center for Health Administration Studies and the Graduate School of Business. We in the center were also wary, but we were willing to test the water, and the dean supported us—a little reluctantly.

A regional meeting for prospective applicants was held by NCHSR representatives in Chicago on March 20, 1975. Universities from the Midwest region sent representatives. The NCHSR was aware of the doubts that we at the University of Chicago had about its new policy of having rather close working relationships with any university-based research center that might be funded. At this conference, the dean spoke quite skeptically about the new policy. Would this attitude jeopardize our chance of having our proposal accepted?

We prepared a very elaborate proposal, enlisting the School of Social Service Administration and relevant departments of the Division of Biological and Social Sciences (the biological sciences embracing the hospitals, clinics, and medical schools). The Mayo Clinic was interested in tying in with us as a delivery system. The clinic already had a health services research unit, which I had visited a few times. In fact, the associate director had previously flown down from Rochester, Minnesota, weekly to attend my course on cross-national comparisons and health policy. We also worked out an arrangement with the Marshfield Clinic in Marshfield, Wisconsin, of a similar type to Mayo. A few years previously, I had been called in by the Marshfield Clinic to advise on the clinic's establishing a health services research unit there. We also had actual and potential working relationships with delivery systems in the Chicago metropolitan area we could tap. Our proposal became a very large and complicated package, which we believed met the not-too-clear guidelines of NCHSR. We were told that the guidelines were negotiable.

In the summer of 1975, NCHSR requested that we present a full-dress rehearsal of our proposal at the University of Chicago, with all collaborators present. The budget had not yet been determined but was to be negotiated later, if we were approved. A representative of NCHSR, Daniel Fox, was there. The day was an exhausting one for me, choreographing the participants and myself to sell the proposal as well as possible. This meeting gave us more visibility in the University of Chicago than before. It appeared to us that we had "pulled it off"—but we were not one of the universities selected for the research-center concept.

Cross-National Activities

I was spending a month to three months every fall in the United Kingdom and Sweden, beginning in 1958, gathering precollected data and official publications on the health services in these two countries (in addition to my similar research in the United States). I came to the realization in the mid 1960s that I needed to get some qualitative impressions through fairly systematic interviews of selected informants in health services administration, politics, labor unions, and academia on the issues they felt were key ones in their respective health services. I spent the major part of my time interviewing informants in Sweden in the fall of 1966 and in Great Britain in 1967. By this time, I had developed a wide network of collegial contacts in both countries. I was fortunate in each country to obtain a prestigious base from which to make appointments for interviews. In Sweden, in the fall of 1966, I worked out of the office of the Department of Social Medicine, University of Uppsala. Bjorn Smedby, in the Department of Social Medicine, helped me find appropriate individuals, mostly in Stockholm, to interview. He had his office call forty to fifty people, to state my mission and arrange interviews. I lived in a hotel in Uppsala and commuted to Stockholm frequently. No one refused to be interviewed, and all were very cordial and open in their answers to my questions. I found that Swedes would talk about any subject with anyone at any time, day or night. They were very flexible and accommodating. Almost all were fluent in English, although at times it was helpful to break over to an occasional Swedish word. I read and understand Swedish because of my Norwegian. In a little more than three weeks, I had completed my interviews. I did not tape them but took notes and elaborated on them as soon as possible later.

In Great Britain, mostly in the London area but also in Manchester, Birmingham, and Edinburgh, I again interviewed forty to fifty counterparts of the Swedes. In London, I was given a desk in the headquarters of the Nuffield Provincial Hospital Trust, counseled by Gordon McLachlan, the director. In the United Kingdom, the pace of bureaucratic life seemed more slow than in Sweden, and the style of arranging interviews was different. Instead of using the telephone, I wrote letters to people whose names had been suggested by McLachlan and others. I got the impression that a letter in longhand on Nuffield stationery would make a better impression than an impersonal telephone call out of the blue. I also discovered that, unlike the Swedes, the British were more ceremonial in setting up interviews, in terms of time and place—never outside working hours, unless for dinner. Clubs were frequent sites for interviews.

Astonishingly (to an American), my letters were answered promptly. This process took me six or more weeks in the United Kingdom, compared to three or so weeks in Sweden. I wrote to Enoch Powell, a Conservative in the House of Commons, for an interview because he had strong views on the National Health Insurance (not to mention views on immigrants from colonies with very different cultures, who were not assimilating well into mainstream British society). He wrote back, and we later had a remarkably congenial, candid, and informative conference, for over an hour.

After 1967, I began to work on my book in earnest, trying to write a comparative history of health services evolution in three countries. It was like three-dimensional chess to synthesize chronologically and cross-sectionally the experiences of three countries. For a while, I thought I could not pull it off; but, after almost ten years of preparation, the material began to fall into place, and a book finally emerged. Like all authors, I was in some suspense about how my book would be received. I had not written it for a special audience, such as medical sociologists and economists, but for the intelligent layperson—health policymakers, hospital administrators, physicians, and so on. This book was the first cross-national comparison study of its kind (Anderson, 1972). I was breaking new ground. I was gratified, of course, that the book was reviewed favorably by a cross-section of interests in both scholarly and interest-group journals. This was more than an author can reasonably expect. I have always been conscious of my relatively nondisciplinary research style, in order to reach a larger reading public.

Between the publication of that book and 1989, I worked on a book to expand the number of liberal-democratic countries covered from three to seven. I selected the countries according to an impressionistic continuum, from highly centralized funding and control to very decentralized: England, Sweden, Canada, West Germany, France, Australia, and the United States. I wrote short histories of each one, showing the evolution of health services and policy in the context of each country. I tried to show what were generic problems that had to be lived with and what were problems that could be solved (Anderson, 1989).

U.S.S.R., September 1972

I was interested in spending some time in the U.S.S.R., to get at least a glimpse of and a feeling for its health services establishment. Reports I had read showed it to be centrally planned, directed, and financed—a quite monolithic structure. Among the Western liberal democracies, the British system approached the U.S.S.R. model.

When President Richard Nixon took office in 1969 he reestablished relationships between the U.S.S.R. and U.S.A. by paying an official visit to that country to revive the various scientific and cultural exchanges that had become moribund. One of the consequences of his visit was a reactivation of exchanges of medical research and health services delivery teams. Early in 1970, Robert Daniels, a professor of psychiatry at the University of Chicago, and I decided to team up and apply to the U.S.S.R.-U.S.A. Exchange Office of the federal government for a traveling fellowship to the

U.S.S.R. and its ministry of health. The director of that office said that we were qualified to be sponsored by this exchange arrangement, and his office would start negotiations. (The word *negotiations* is used advisedly because exchange of any kind between the U.S.A. and the U.S.S.R. at that time could be slow.) The standard arrangement was that the U.S. government paid expenses to Moscow, and the Soviet government paid for all other expenses. The arrangement was very official and formal.

We and the Exchange Office waited a year and a half for word from the ministry of health of the U.S.S.R. The Exchange Office had been unable to get any reply. The spring of 1972 was approaching, and Daniels and I needed to plan for the fall. (By this time, Daniels had moved to Cincinnati.) I finally called the director of the Exchange Office and said that I had to make plans. He said he would call the ministry of health in the U.S.S.R. immediately and find out what was going on. A couple of days later he called back and said, "You are in. The ministry will accept your visit during the month of June or September 1972." We said we preferred the month of September; I could then time the U.S.S.R. trip with my annual trip to northern Europe.

Daniels and I were flown to Washington, D.C., for a briefing. We were told that both the American Embassy and the ministry of health in Moscow had been notified that we would arrive on Aerflot from London on September 6 at 6 P.M. The custom was that a representative of the ministry would meet us at the airport, take us to our hotel, and help us get started on our visit. Further, to my astonishment, I was asked to look into the possibility of negotiating a contract between the ministry of health and the U.S. Department of Health, Education, and Welfare (HEW) to study the nature and operation of the U.S.S.R. health services. The health services appeared to be a secret at that time, not normally open to study by foreigners. This suggestion, of course, fit neatly into my cross-national interests.

We were flown to London and, with a short layover, boarded the Aerflot flight nonstop to Moscow. We landed in Moscow in the dark. Neither Daniels nor I knew any Russian. What would we do if no one was there to meet us? We got off the plane and were expeditiously put through customs and immigration, for we were designated as VIPs. We strolled into the waiting room. Almost immediately, a smartly dressed woman (suit and black boots) approached us and asked in very correct English if we were Professors Anderson and Daniels. I was so relieved that I paternally put my arm around her and said, "Here we are." I saw an office window, which I took for a bank, and I said I wished to cash an American Express check. She said "On no, I have money for you for two days, until the ministry of health gives you your allowance for the month." I said to myself, "So, this is Communism. I was never treated like this in Washington." She hailed a taxicab, and we took off and registered at a cavernous prerevolutionary European-type hotel. We were taken to a comfortable two-room suite with bath, television, and radio.

Next morning, our guide met us at the hotel and took us by subway to the ministry. A doctor in his early thirties took us over with courtesy and gusto. He had just returned from an exchange-program trip from the United States himself. He spoke fluent English. He said that since we were going to be in the U.S.S.R. for a whole month, he had not yet planned anything for us. After he knew what we wanted to see, the program could be quickly planned. We said we were after information, data, and statistics on the operation of the health service and were less interested in visiting a whole string of hospitals and clinics. He caught on quickly and said that we should spend a great deal of our time with personnel in the Shemoshko Institute in Moscow. This institute was the data-collection and research arm of the ministry of health. We would visit hospitals and clinics in Moscow and the institute for three weeks and then spend the last week in Leningrad, on our way home. All in all, we were cordially received by all the highly placed people in the health services and given a great deal of oral and printed information. On occasion, I brought up the possibility of a contract between their ministry and our HEW. The technical people, the statisticians, were interested in cooperating, but the higher up we got into the hierarchy, the less expression of interest there was. My impression was that the exchange program was based on reciprocal interests, and that there was no interest in health services of the United States. The Soviets already had the delivery structure they wanted and would not learn anything. What they wanted to learn about was medical technology, which they felt was deficient in the U.S.S.R. (Anderson, 1973).

What I got out of that visit to the U.S.S.R. was a feeling for a very different style of organizing and running a health service. It was a command system; the West is characterized by a demand system.

The last week of September we spent in Leningrad, hosted by the health authorities in that city. We were met at the railroad station by a psychiatrist from the Pavlov Institute and an interpreter. (We had two interpreters during that week, who were graduate students in American literature at the University of Leningrad.)

While in Leningrad, we met a party of American psychiatrists, led by a physician from the National Institute of Mental Health, Washington, D.C. He told me why our application had been held up so long by the Soviet Embassy in Washington. A Soviet in that embassy whom he had come to know well called him up and asked if he knew somebody by the name of Odin Anderson. The American said that he knew me quite well. The Russian said that he could not make out my political orientation from my curriculum vitae. He asked if I was an appropriate person to be admitted into the U.S.S.R. on this exchange program. The Soviet government could accept or reject any person proposed by the U.S. government, and the reverse was also true. The American leader said that I was a well-respected health services researcher and was not known for any political activities or words of that nature. I was then cleared.

What struck me about the U.S.S.R. health services was the lavish supply of medical personnel of various specialties and the many types of specialists. Generalists as such were not recognized. Even primary-care physicians—first-entry physicians, almost all women—were called specialists. What also struck me was the specialization among institutions: hospitals for adults, hospitals for children (under seventeen), hospitals for maternity services (but, less surprising, hospitals and day-care centers for the mentally ill). The emergency services were also separate, with fleets of ambulances. There were outpatient departments for each of the specialty hospitals. Each institutional type had its own catchment area. The first entry point was the primary physician for each specialty hospital.

Each institution had its own variety of specialists. There was little or no overlap of physicians. By Western standards, this system was inefficient and uncoordinated; by Western standards (which may not necessarily be an appropriate reference point), the utilization rate was high (ten visits per physician per capita), compared with Western rates of three.

After an afternoon in an adult outpatient department, I noticed in the waiting room a wall full of cubicles containing the records of patients who had appointments that day. At the end of the time, the staff knew who had not come.

"Then what do you do?" I asked.

"We go and get them or call them."

Australia, October 1976

Early in 1976, I had a telegram from the Australian Hospital Association, inviting me to attend its two-day annual conference in Sydney and give the keynote address in October of the same year. In addition, I would be hosted for twelve days, to confer with anyone in Australia who was well connected with Australia's health service and health insurance program. The association would make the appointments and fly me wherever the informants might be. I would be flown first-class from Chicago to Sydney and return. Naturally, this was an easy offer to accept.

Somewhat boldly, I wrote back and said that normally I was in northern Europe before the Australian visit was scheduled. Instead of my returning to Chicago and flying to Australia, would the association buy a tourist-class around-the-world ticket, which would cost no more than the round-trip Chicago–Sydney first-class ticket? A return telegram said yes, as long as the tourist-class fare was not more than a first-class fare. I then planned to fly to Sydney from London via Kabul, Afghanistan, and Delhi, India, and stop for a couple of days in each place. I had never been there. (My wife and daughter had traveled from London to Istanbul, Turkey, to Nepal and back to Israel and Chicago in February of the same year. They insisted I stop in Kabul, at least. Given the awful events in Kabul not long after my visit, I am, of course, glad I did.)

The twelve days in Australia are one of the most memorable

trips I have ever taken. The hospitality was friendly and lavish. I learned a great deal about the Australian health services and the vacillating policy on whether to have universal health insurance or not. I had read up on the Australian health services, to the extent that there was any literature on it, and got many insights from people in politics, administration, and academia. It was not enough that I gave two addresses at the annual conference of the Australian Hospital Association; I also held seminars at Monash University in Melbourne and in the Department of Health and Welfare of the state of New South Wales, in Sydney.

Australia was a complete contrast to the U.S.S.R., with characteristics very close to those of the United States, but at that time more pluralistic and private. Public subsidies for premiums for physicians' insurance and for hospital care were used to maintain a semblance of private enterprise, to avoid complete governmental control. Australia had been going through rather chaotic policy debates and implementation of the policy for universal health insurance, which has stabilized only recently. Australia now has a mixed public-private health insurance program, with three options: complete public, with no choice of specialist; public, with choice of specialist at a higher price; or completely private, with open choice of private insurance. The latter is obligatory. The Australian Medical Association is even more intransigent than the American Medical Association and has been able to maintain the standard private-practice fee-for-service system, contracting with the government and insurance companies.

A Mediterranean Cruise

In 1975, I was approached by the Louisiana Medical Society and the Medical Society of St. Louis, Missouri, which had chartered a ship for a twelve-day cruise in the Mediterranean in October 1975. These were the days when the Internal Revenue Service permitted professional groups to take a tour during which they could engage professors to give lectures on board ship on subjects relevant to professional groups (in this case, physicians). These lectures were defined as continuing education, and the tour expenses were tax-exempt. I was invited to give four lectures, and all expenses for my wife and me were paid. Naturally, we had to accept this generous offer.

The Greek cruise ship was comfortable and lavish, with excellent food. We started from Athens and went ashore in Alexandria and Cairo. We went on to Haifa, Israel; to the island of Rhodes; and to Ephesus, on the Turkish coast. In Alexandria and Haifa, physicians came aboard to tell the cruise physicians about their respective health services.

I was asked to lecture on the status of health services organization and finance in the United States, which would perforce deal with the question of government health insurance. In the first lecture, I began to outline the issues in government health insurance and the prevailing private health insurance in the United States. There were around seventy-five physicians in the audience. I began to note a sense of hostility from the audience. People did not seem to like what they were hearing. I was simply, in usual academic fashion, describing the issues and what was taking place and making some tentative predictions for the near future. The physicians were a conservative lot. I confronted them and said, "Do not kill the messenger on the first day of this cruise. You invited me to give lectures on this subject, and I want to enjoy the whole cruise, as you do." This broke the ice completely, and they were a friendly bunch thereafter. I remember particularly a general surgeon from southern Illinois befriending me as a symbolic act for his colleagues.

Postscript

In 1980, when I retired from the University of Chicago, Ronald Andersen became director of the Center for Health Administration Studies. I continued my own research from my positions at the University of Chicago and the University of Wisconsin–Madison.

Andersen, with his staff, engaged in a great deal of research from 1980 to 1990, maintaining the momentum of the previous decade by developing and expanding his own research interests within the general framework that he had helped me establish from the time I appointed him, in 1963, until 1980. I do not intend to make a detailed review of the research projects and publications by him and his staff, but to give some idea of the scope of their research, which continued after I was no longer director. Andersen was generous in calling me a consultant on the projects that he and his staff promoted.

Andersen, in essence, moved into evaluation research and its methodology, directed to the degree to which contemporary health insurance was equalizing access to health services according to income level, residence (inner cities), and race. He and his staff devised a severity index of access to services, demonstrating that although the gap between use of services and family income was converging over time, standardization for severity of symptoms revealed that lower-income groups had more severe symptoms than upper-income groups did. The lower-income groups were less likely to seek care for less severe symptoms but still should seek care for them, compared with upper-income groups. Other studies moved into evaluations of particular programs, such as primary freestanding physician-care adjuncts to hospitals and home care for ventilator-assisted children. The book-length reports were published, as well as many articles on the health services from a cross-disciplinary perspective in economics, behavioral science, and political science.

The following publications are illustrative: Aday, Fleming, and Andersen (1984), Aday, Andersen, Loevy, and Kremer (1985), Aday, Aitken, and Wegener (1988), and Fleming and Andersen (1986). The funding for the research during the 1980s came from the Division of Maternal and Child Health of the U.S. Department of Health and Human Resources and from the Robert Wood Johnson Foundation. Ronald Andersen and his staff are now working on the first cross-national survey of dental programs and practices in fourteen countries, including eastern Europe and the U.S.S.R. The major funding is from the World Health Organization, which, along with Andersen, coordinates the survey.

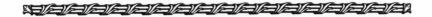

8

The University
of Wisconsin–Madison,
1980–1990

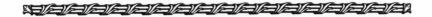

In 1979, I was approaching the compulsory retirement age of sixty-five at the University of Chicago. My sixty-fifth birthday fell on July 5. The rule permitted a faculty member to finish the fiscal year, which was July 1 to July 1, no matter at what point his or her birthday fell. This meant that I had, in effect, an extra year. The dean of the Graduate School of Business called me late in 1978 and asked if I was aware of this. I said that I was. I was really ready to retire, if the atmosphere in the dean's office indicated that I was expected to retire. When the dean knew that I knew I had an extra year, he said, "That is terrific." So I remained until July 1, 1980.

In the fall of 1979, I was all set to move to Madison in the summer of 1980 to retire. My wife and I had planned for years to retire to Madison, our old stamping ground. We already owned a house near the campus, which we had bought in 1971 in anticipation of moving there after retirement.

During my last year at the University of Chicago, the Graduate School of Business and I were trying to find a successor to me as director of the Center for Health Administration Studies and of the program in hospital administration. As was the criterion at the university, a successor had to be a scholar and have administrative ability. Ronald Andersen was a reluctant candidate. He did not wish to erode the valuable time for research he was enjoying. He was in the same situation I was in 1970, when Bugbee retired. We found no suitable candidate who would be interested. Nevertheless, Ronald Andersen agreed to succeed me. He inherited rather good financial resources to work with. We still had the reserve funds that Bugbee and I had brought with us from New York in 1962, and he had the ability to raise research money on his own.

I had decided prior to my retirement not to look for or expect anything. I would move to Madison and be near extensive library and cultural resources. I also had a sixty-acre farm in the hills of western Wisconsin, only a few miles from where I grew up and from the village where I went to high school. I would engage in the history of Norwegian immigrants. In 1925, a professional historical society called the Norwegian-American Historical Association had been established, which published articles and books. I would learn how to play the piano again.

When colleagues in sociology and history at the University of Wisconsin learned that I was moving to Madison, I was privileged to be asked if I would be interested in a half-time teaching appointment in the department until I turned seventy, the University of Wisconsin's retirement age. The emerging Program in Health Services Administration in the medical school was also interested in my move to Madison. The head of the Department of Sociology, then Aage Sorensen, began discussions with me. Then the dean of the Graduate School of Business of the University of Chicago offered me a three-year contract full-time, with no administrative duties. (Ronald Andersen told him he wanted me around.) I told the dean that I was contemplating an academic post at the University of Wisconsin half-time, and if appropriate details were ironed out, I would accept. He then offered me a half-time appointment as professor emeritus for three years.

In the meantime, Sorensen was trying to devise suitable titles. I said that if I was going to help medical sociology at Wisconsin, I would have to have a title, so that I could talk to generals. He tried "visiting professor." I said, "It sounds too temporary." I asked if I would have a guaranteed four-year contract, so that I could be assured of continuity in whatever I wanted to develop at Wisconsin. He said that a letter of agreement would be sufficient. A month or so passed. Finally, he called me up and said, "You have been appointed a professor with tenure, half-time, until your seventieth birthday." I accepted both positions at the two universities. I asked the dean of letters and science at Wisconsin if he would mind my also teaching at the University of Chicago. "No problem," he said. I asked the same of the dean at the University of Chicago: "No problem." (At this writing, in July 1990, I have completed ten years of commuting between Madison and Chicago and have terminated teaching at Chicago.)

To backtrack to the last year I was at the University of Chicago, Bernard Nelson, vice-president of the Henry J. Kaiser Family Foundation, in Menlo Park, California, wanted to see me early in 1979. The Kaiser Foundation was looking for academic sites that could administer scholarships for students in schools of business and management who were interested in health services administration. The foundation wanted to attract the best students by offering quite generous scholarships. I took him to see the dean. Nelson stated his mission. The dean asked what sort of money was being contemplated. Nelson said some figure around $500,000. The dean, instead of being impressed, said the school would ask for $1 million. I thought we would lose the whole deal with that rejoinder; but, in due course, the school, on behalf of its Program in Health Administration, received this amount and more.

I asked Nelson if there could also be a grant for research. I told him that I had been making some exploratory investigations in Minneapolis–St. Paul regarding the rapid emergence of HMOs in competition with one another and with the mainstream fee-for-service system. The market penetration of the HMOs was then approaching 20 percent of the population of two million people in the Twin Cities metropolitan area. Here was an opportunity to analyze the social and political environment in which the HMOs developed: the business and industrial base, the political context, the nature of the market, the medical practice and referral patterns of physicians, the use of hospitals, and the selection characteristics of people enrolled in HMOs and in the mainstream health services system.

Nelson said there were many rumors and anecdotes emanating from the Twin Cities area, and a good study would help to set the record straight. I said that there was now adequate enough research methodology in organizations, health services, and consumer behavior so that, in a three-year period, it would be possible to reveal what was going on in the Twin Cities area, historically and currently. Nelson was enthusiastic about this research prospect. He indicated that the foundation was looking around for good and relevant research projects (relevant to public policy). I said this project would not be cheap; it might approach $3 million. He seemed to accept that and proposed that I move ahead and formulate a project, including the elements just listed. I said that I would need some start-up money because working up a research project involves a lot of staff time. I also suggested that this project was big and complex enough that I would need to approach the health services research unit at the School of Public Health, University of Minnesota, to collaborate with us. What did I need? I said $25,000. He agreed, and in due time this start-up grant was provided.

I immediately went to Minneapolis, to confer with my research colleagues in the School of Public Health. The project was too big for one research center. The reception was enthusiastic. My staff and I had several sessions in Minneapolis, mapping out the division of labor in relation to our respective interests and research skills. In a rather short time, we worked out an elaborate but feasible research protocol with a piece for all of us and a budget for each piece, shared between us and our School of Public Health collaborators. For myself, I carved out the project dealing with the history of the development of the HMO concept in the Twin Cities and Minnesota and its sociopolitical context. Some of the data would be found in already existing records. Additional data, adding flesh to the bare bones of statistical information, would be obtained in extensive personal interviews with informants in the Twin Cities area: physicians, business and industry leaders, regulators, and insurance and HMO administrators. The total budget exceeded $2 million for three years, allocated to the various projects. My project was set at $80,000.

Representatives from the School of Public Health and from CHAS at the University of Chicago were flown to the California headquarters of the Kaiser Foundation to present our project before the president and staff of the foundation, including Nelson. The willingness of the foundation to host us seemed to be a good sign that the proposal would be accepted. We made our presentation. Those present appeared to be impressed but made no commitment. The proposal would be presented to the board of the foundation in the very near future. The board rejected it. My historical-development project on the sociopolitical environment of the HMOs was accepted, however, with the budget proposed ($80,000). Our disappointment was keen. Nelson was quite crushed because, as a rather new vice-president, he thought he was backing something significant and big (and he was).

I assembled an excellent staff of four, all graduate students at the University of Chicago in sociology and business (except one, who was working on a Ph.D. dissertation from Michigan State University; she was in Chicago because her dissertation dealt with an early HMO in the Chicago area, and her husband, a pediatrician, took over a children's hospital near the university and had an academic post in the Department of Pediatrics). We then conceived of the idea of including the Chicago metropolitan area, in order to compare HMO developments between the Twin Cities and Chicago, two markedly different market and urban areas. By this time (1980), the HMOs in Chicago had penetrated only 3 percent of the market. We scrounged around for money to finance the Chicago-area research. We got enough money, just barely, from the Chicago Community Trust, the Blue Cross–Blue Shield plan of Illinois. The Blue plans already had begun to foster HMOs. The Kaiser Family Foundation also supported part of the costs of the Chicago project. It took until the end of 1981 and early 1982 to get the project started in both urban areas. Our access to the Twin Cities' health services establishment was easy. All parties concerned were hospitable.

Our access to the Chicago-area establishment took a little longer. The HMOs in the area were skeptical. There were eight struggling HMOs in Chicago at that time, in a population of seven million. (There were seven in the Twin Cities, with a population of two million.) The Chicago HMOs had a federation of HMOs, including those outside Chicago. They were wary of being studied at this early stage of their growth. I asked permission to present our project to a regular meeting of the federation. It was granted. The president of the federation was sympathetic. After my presentation, the members voted acceptance as a federation, but individual HMOs could accept being studied or not. We gained entry to all, although one of them required some persistence. The director said he had had some bad experiences with researchers and reporters. Entry to that

HMO was finally granted because I was trusted as an objective researcher.

While the Twin Cities–Chicago HMO research program was going into operation, I moved to Madison, in July 1980. (My wife had moved ahead of me, in 1974, and so I already had an established hearth.) I supervised the Twin Cities–Chicago project from my continuing research base at the University of Chicago and from Madison. Early in September, I joined the faculty of the Department of Sociology and the faculty of the Program in Health Services Administration at the University of Wisconsin–Madison. At the University of Chicago, I was appointed half-time on July 1, 1980. In the fall, I began teaching at both universities.

The research areas were divided among the staff, according to their competence and interest: the hospitals, physicians, regulatory agencies, HMOs, and the market characteristics. I brooded, one might say, over the whole enterprise and worked on the historical and political context of the emergence of the HMOs. We interviewed influential people in the Twin Cities area, selected according to their positions in the foregoing areas. Appointments were made from the Chicago base—a horrendous telephone activity. Many of the informants were hard to reach the first time. We set aside three days at a time to assemble in Minneapolis and fan out for interviews, four of us doing around four a day. The foregoing was repeated in the Chicago area. We conducted about 150 interviews in each area. All the interviews were partially focused and open-ended. All were taped. (Only one person in St. Paul refused to be taped; the interviewee was a state civil servant.) Interviews took about an hour, on the average. The informants were frank.

The project took from 1980 until 1984 to complete. I had assumed that all of the data would be given to me in organized form, and I would do the major synthesis of writing, as I had done in previous projects. This time, however, the staff wanted to write the chapters relevant to their own work themselves, and I would tie them together with introductory and closing chapters. I agreed, having faith that the writing would be sufficiently uniform in style. Each author would be identified in the chapters each prepared. It worked. The chapters were gratifyingly uniform. I was spared a tremendous writing job.

Before publication of the report, we held a public meeting in Minneapolis for all who were involved, to present our major findings. It went well. Later, we had a public meeting in Chicago, in connection with our annual Symposium on Hospital Affairs. That meeting also went well. In 1985, the report was published in full (Anderson and others, 1985).

We were reluctant to let the project stop at this point. In Minneapolis–St. Paul particularly, the HMOs and the mainstream fee-for-service models were beginning to clash as the big employer market was being saturated. The Twin Cities were approaching a mature market stage, which was beginning to change the health services establishment, affecting hospitals and physicians' practices, not to mention consumers. We believed that we now knew the major variables to monitor the changes taking place in the Twin Cities' health services establishment. We approached the Kaiser Foundation for more funds to continue to study this unique situation—a live laboratory, right before our eyes. The foundation, however, was no longer interested in HMOs. I got the impression that the foundation president and staff felt that HMOs were now on their way, and the foundation could turn to other cutting-edge problems, such as quality control and health and life-style relationships. This was now 1984–1985, and I was completing five years of teaching, research, and commuting between Madison and Chicago, making a trip a week for two days, up to thirty weeks a year. Summers were free.

In 1984, I was approaching my seventieth birthday. My understanding with the University of Wisconsin was that I would retire, as was the regulation at that university. The custom was very rigid there that no one was rehired after age seventy. One day, late in 1983, the head of the department, Gerald Marwell, had burst into my office. He had been going over the new appointments, resignations, and retirements of the sociology faculty for the coming fiscal year. He had reported to the university personnel office that I was due to retire on June 30, 1984. The personnel office said "not true" because my birthday fell at the beginning of the fiscal year, and the regulation was that, in effect, I had another year, if I wanted to stay on. The head of the department grinned and asked if I wanted to stay on. I said, "Yes." I was repeating my University of Chicago experience. As the fates would have it, that same year the Wisconsin legislature passed a law that no employer could release an employee only because of age, including university professors. I had, in effect, been granted life tenure. It is now 1990, and I am still teaching.

The HMO study became my last large-scale research project, and I was ready to feel relieved. Nevertheless, I would have relished setting up a long-term project monitoring the dynamics of the Twin Cities' HMOs and mature market developments. If this had come to pass, I could have found others to take the supervisory duties.

Concurrently with research and teaching, I was always assembling and organizing data on the development of the American health services and, similarly, on the European countries I was visiting annually. I wanted to rewrite and update a book I had published in 1968, which was a history of the American health services from 1875 to 1965, making some revisions and bringing the history up to the beginning of the Reagan administration. I also wanted to rewrite another of my books (Anderson, 1972). I wanted to include four more liberal-democratic countries, for a more linear continuum than was attempted in the earlier book. The revision and updating of the history of the American health services was eventually published (Anderson, 1985).

After finishing the book on the history of the American health services, I started in earnest on the new book on cross-national comparisons of health services. I would include more countries among liberal-democratic states, in order to have a continuum of countries, from centralized to decentralized systems, among other variables. My primary purpose would be to demonstrate what could be done with preexisting data from seven countries, to understand how they evolved, what were the political and social issues within each country that led to action for health insurance, what seemed to account for the different configurations of organizational and financing differences, and what were the aggregate and gross differences in expenditures, supply, and use of services. The book would be an overview of cross-national research and what can be generalized from that base about the nature of health services in developed liberal-democratic countries.

A contract was executed with the publisher—with, presumably, a mutual understanding of the style I was going to use. There was a great deal of further assembling and organization of information and data on the three countries I had covered in my book in 1972—the United States, Sweden, and England. I had to start from scratch for the other countries—Canada, France, West Germany, and Australia—although I had a great deal of material piled up in my office, collected over twenty years. In addition, given my network of contacts in all the countries mentioned, I had good informants who conscientiously sent me recent official publications and studies on request.

By 1987, I had completed the final draft. There had been a change in staff at the publisher, and the previous health editor had been replaced. I met the new editor in New York to review what I understood had been agreed on with the previous editor. She had not yet seen any part of the manuscript, but what I discussed with her appeared to be acceptable.

I sent the manuscript to the editor. A few weeks later, I had a letter that expressed great disappointment with the manuscript. She had expected a textbook, but what she got was, in her judgment, a lot of "opinions." It seemed that the shift in personnel had also resulted in a shift in policy. I said that the so-called opinions were interpretations, based on as much information and insight as possible, given the state of the art. Cross-national comparisons of health services delivery systems were not yet ready for textbook presentation. This was a conceptual book, trying to show where more primary research was necessary, beyond preexisting information and data. Obviously, we were at odds, and we agreed to rescind the contract. I would retain my manuscript, to do with as I pleased.

While this exchange was going on, the Health Administration Press, which had published a previous book of mine, learned about it through the publishers' grapevine. The editor wrote me a letter, expressing interest in the manuscript and indicating that she wished to review it for publication by her press. She recognized that the topic was timely, I had long experience in cross-national research, and my previous book was selling well. I submitted the manuscript, and after a short review period the manuscript was accepted, with mutual agreement about revisions, expansions, and shortening—the usual process between author and publisher. The book was published in 1989 (Anderson, 1989).

On top of this, the Health Administration Press wanted an update of my history of the American health services through the Reagan administration, which I did in the summer of 1989. I was very pleased to have this request, because I felt (as the Press did) that my earlier book was somewhat unfinished because ferment in the health field was not yet taking on a pattern that would predict how the health field would look by 1990. This is not to say that the 1990s will become crystal clear, but the trends are becoming much clearer.

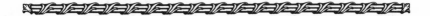

9

Lessons for Applied Social Science Researchers

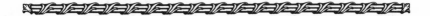

What can be learned from the foregoing chapters? The first piece of advice is "Know thyself." Learn to know the substantive content of any institution, enterprise, or program more thoroughly than any one of your informants. My own experience has been in the macro characteristics of health services delivery systems. A risk you run in becoming thoroughly involved in studying an enterprise is to be co-opted, to begin to think too much like the enterprise and people you study. Therefore, "Know thyself," so that you can maintain enough detachment. Some degree of co-optation is quite functional. You must assume and be comfortable with a marginal role, being inside the enterprise you study but not of it.

As will be recalled from the early chapters, those who regarded themselves as social scientists with a mission to improve society had a subliminal belief in a natural moral order, which governed the good society, how society could be improved, and what the characteristics of such a society were. It was a society without crime and poverty, one in which there was full citizen participation in a liberal-democratic political process and freedom of speech, assembly, and the press, to facilitate discussion based on objective facts. There was belief in education for everybody. There was belief in creating a meritocracy, based on individual merit and the effort of a circulating elite, replacing hereditary ones. The good society was the result of good people, who, because they were good, created good institutions (now called "capitalism with a human face"). Even the Great Depression of the 1930s, World War II and its horrors, and the Cold War did not essentially weaken this view among the older generation (including myself) that experienced them. After World War II, a new generation of social scientists was trained who, by and large, rejected this individualistic view of society. Instead, the generally accepted wisdom was that existing society itself created the bad social conditions of crime and poverty. The problems were systemic, not individual. Society needed to be reformed, which in turn would result in good people.

Among social science academics, a primary method of trying to create a good society was social research on the festering social problems— setting forth their dimensions and the apparent causes. Facts would suggest self-evident solutions. This is almost a caricature, but not quite; social scientists' experiences described in the foregoing chapters seem to support this observation. The political process, rather than being an orderly process of negotiation and compromise among interest groups, would be a product of social research—in short, a product of technocrats, which would be agreed to by all reasonable people, or at least a large enough majority to override the unreasonable minority and neutralize it politically.

The generation of social scientists who engaged in applied social research after World War II—and, particularly, beginning during the Kennedy administration, in 1962, and continuing into the Reagan administration, in the 1980s—produced an abundance of applied research results in the health services and general welfare, too extensive to be listed here. During the latter 1960s into the 1980s, a rather extensive and thoughtful literature appeared, written by social scientists who examined the very idea of applied research, its relevance to policy, the problems of gaining access to programs and institutions as detached observers interested in policy-related research, and the problem of their own values. Many of these researchers (Deitchman, Glazer, Grant, Haveman, Horowitz, Lee, Moynihan, Nielsen, Pettigrew and Green, Rainwater and Yancy) have been cited in previous chapters. Others are listed in Selected Readings, a resource section that follows Chapter Ten.

There was a surge of research during the Kennedy and Johnson administrations, quickly followed by evaluations of this research for public policy. The optimism among many social scientists—that applied social research would be of major help in improving society through the War on Poverty and in improving education for blacks (through busing, for example)—was blunted by the failure of the Johnson administration to turn society around toward the anticipated "brave new world." A "taking stock" literature emerged, a literature that now began to recognize that social scientists do not know enough about social processes, how society ticks, to be able to guide society sufficiently to eliminate poverty and to bring blacks and low-income segments into the mainstream middle-class level of standards and accomplishments; there were too many unintended consequences and latent functions. A social-engineering mentality prevailed, trying to emulate the physical sciences in going to the moon (as remarked by one sage commentator during this period, "We got to the moon because there were no people between it and the earth"). The social scientists began to recognize that social research was only one of the factors, and not even an independent variable, in the political process of formulating public policy. They had to begin to think politically as well as technically, as an integral part of the process of policy formulation. In fact, several social scientists seriously doubted that scientists should be on top as philosopher kings, but on tap. A social scientist's values regarding the good society are no better or worse than the values espoused by the representatives of the people (the elected politicians) or the range of interest groups, as long as they operate within a liberal-democratic political-process framework.

Some writers doubted that social scientists should ever, as scientists, make explicit recommendations on means and ends. They do not know enough about the relationship between the two, although they certainly carry ideals in their heads of the good society. Perhaps the best that social scientists can do is to advise on whether a certain means can result in a desired end and, in so doing, give, say, three options. The implementers then have to take it from there. Demographers, for example, eventually got around to predicting population growth, deaths, and births by offering high, medium, and low trends, given certain assumptions. I wish to make it clear that social scientists, as citizens, can espouse any policies they wish but should not presume that such policies are attainable, given current knowledge. One writer asserted that democracy should be allowed to make egregious mistakes, a learning process in itself.

In this context, there was a realization that on hindsight seems naïve: social scientists were surprised by how difficult it is to reform society. The necessary reforms seemed to be self-evident to all reasonable people, but the intervening interest groups were inclined to maintain the status quo and strive for incremental rather than quick reform. Thus, one writer observed that applied social science research was possibly a conservative influence in itself because such research many times showed how intractable so many of the social problems were. I have felt this way many times myself as a liberal, and increasingly so as I got older. I have come to the reluctant conclusion that I am an "empirical conservative." The evidence induces that position.

Some social scientists behave more like moral philosophers than empirical social scientists. For example, there are now very good bioethicists who ponder the ethics of abortions, life prolongation, how to ration justly with scarce medical resources, and so on. They help to clarify the decision-making process in adopting one ethical stand or another.

The social scientists are so fragmented that we join social-policy "think tanks" trying to rationalize either liberal policies or conservative policies and to decide to what degree public policies should be implemented through government or through the market. The Brookings Institution, on the liberal side, and the American Enterprise Institute, on the conservative side, are prototypical examples. In fact, policymakers have their choice of legitimate, competent, respectable social scientists to justify contrary policies on the basis of their theories (and, when possible, their empirical work). Compared with standard physics or chemistry, the social sciences are a weird world. When I was research director of the Health Information Foundation, I was a liberal in a conservative context, but a context that supported and had faith in the power of empirical fact. I was thus able to survive and flourish according to my mission.

Some social scientists wrote about the problem of evaluating ongoing social programs (like Head Start), the effects of a negative income-tax demonstration in New Jersey, or the success of efforts to rehabilitate criminals in prisons and reduce recidivism. There was frustration because the program sponsors and administrators were hardly ever given measurable and specific objectives or told what was an acceptable level of attainment. All social welfare and health programs inherently do not make explicit what would be an acceptable level of attainment. The objectives seem to imply a zero-sum game, 100 percent attainment. There appears to be no concept of a socially and politically acceptable level of attainment as to the possible within a certain equilibrium of forces. There is an underlying standard of utopianism. Hospitals, for example, have no acceptable standard for inpatient death rates. Alcohol and drug-addiction programs have no operational concept of reasonable attainment, given all the intractable factors involved. Perhaps the reason is that professionalism assumes always to strive for perfection.

I just said that I regard myself as an empirical conservative. The evidence for that observation is all around us, historically and currently. At the same time, such a view allows for no hope for major improvements in society. Utopian thinkers frighten me because, if they gained power, they would become authoritarians. Still, unless one reaches for the stars, improvements will not take place. Hence, utopian thinkers give me latitude to be "moderate" from either the left or the right. Utopian thinkers are both extreme leftists and extreme rightists. Classical sociologists and classical laissez-faire economists are both utopians. In an operating liberal-democratic society, there is a "vital center" where there can be give-and-take and compromise, within extremes. These extremes give a person like me an opportunity to be able to be an empirical conservative who does not expect too much, given the human condition, but who also runs the danger of expecting too little. After I reached the age of sixty, I believe, I began to tell my students in health policy that when I was young I overestimated the possible; now, I run the danger of underestimating the possible. Energy diminishes. Intransigent problems seem to continue or repeat themselves. Solve one problem, and a different one takes its place in a new context, which creates perceptions of new problems after one appears to be solved. The health field is rife with new problems as old ones are even partially resolved. A case in point is that universal health insurance solves the problem of the cost of expensive services for the individual at the time of service, but when there is resistance to taxation, public policymakers must have priorities within the tax sources available. The universal results are rationing and waiting lists for nonlethal medical conditions.

Another problem dealt with by some writers is the privilege of social scientists to obtain data from institutions and programs. Social scientists expose institutions to their own limitations; "the emperor has no clothes." They assume that they work in the public interest and should expect to be allowed to engage in research on the internal operations, objectives, failures, and attainments of institutions. Social research is not in the same category as investigative journalism; the rules of the game are different. In social research involving institutions, programs, and people, the subjects of research have the right to privacy and to be told precisely what the research objectives are, who the sponsor and the funding sources are, how much the research may interfere with daily operations, and how long the research will take. It is also diplomatic and courteous to have the research report read by appropriate parties who are subjects of the research, for possible errors of fact and interpretation. The researchers, however, must reserve the right to publish, as dictated by their scientific integrity. If the right to publish will not be granted, there can be no research project. All these specifications, to be obvious, must be agreed to by the researchers and the subjects in advance. If it is not possible to obtain mutual trust and respect, it is exceedingly unwise for researchers to proceed.

The foregoing is the academic stance. If the objective and motive of academics is to muckrake or expose "bad" practices, it is not legitimate for them to pose as objective researchers. Obviously, these rules apply mainly when a research design necessitates personal interviews or access to internal records of an institution. Any information in the public domain (newspapers, official reports, statistical reports, and so on) scarcely needs permission to be used. Many social scientists who have conducted research on philanthropic foundations, business operations, academic institutions, and others, limiting themselves to published sources, have come out with some understanding of how institutions function. These macro-level studies may not need information that an institution, for its own reasons, may deem confidential and nobody else's business.

In applied social research, the need for tested methodology cannot be overemphasized. It is in the nature of applied research that the parties at interest will be offended by the results, and the first attack is on the methodology. (This is also true, of course, of research intended to build up a discipline, but there are different consequences and reactions.) Frequently, the results of applied research have practical consequences for a given public policy. (In discipline-oriented research, the consequences are more or less limited to research peers who are interested in building theories and generalizations therefrom.) Therefore, applied researchers, particularly if the results may be socially and politically controversial, should not experiment but should apply only tested and generally accepted methodology. (This is not to say, of course, that tested, tried methodology in applied research may not contribute to the improvement of methodology in general.)

Sociologists are increasingly working in nonacademic settings—marketing and advertising firms, government agencies, trade associations, and professional associations. I know quite a few of them. It can be sensed that they may have problems reconciling the academic professional role, with its freedom to teach, write, and publish, and the professional role in these nonacademic settings. The academic-professional role and its functional privileges are the reference points for social scientists in nonacademic settings.

The very first consideration for social scientists is acceptance of the missions of nonacademic agencies. One person may not approve of working in a birth-control agency; another may feel that it has a legitimate public-interest mission. One person may not want to work for an advertising agency marketing cigarettes; another may feel that people have a right to consume whatever they wish. One person may not want to work in a trade or professional association because of its stand on health issues, and so on. Whatever the mission, it is incumbent on the social scientist to respect it if he or she accepts employment in a particular agency. In turn, the social scientist must perform at professional standards of quality, integrity, honesty, and competence, as any other professional does. One characteristic of all nonacademic institutions is that there is no necessary right to publish in-house research for the institution's own use. Further, the social scientist should expect that an institution may, according to its own policy, request certain types of data gathering or studies that managers feel will be of more use to them than other types. A well-run institution will probably consult the professional researcher on what projects can be of help to the institution, within its mission. The professional researcher must certainly advise the institution on the feasibility of the methodology necessary for data gathering of various kinds.

Researchers in nonacademic institutions largely work *for* the institutions, not *at* them. Conversely, academically based researchers largely work *at* the institutions, not *for* them. For example, people assumed I was working *for* the Health Information Foundation, but I was working *at* the foundation, within the mission of its sponsors, as I understood and agreed with it. Indeed, my stance gave the foundation the credibility in health services research that it sought.

Applied research frequently is of interest to the mass media. The media are a constant problem for social scientists. Given the current "state of the art" in the social sciences, only rarely can social scientists give a completely unequivocal assertion on the evidence. Social scientists have produced an enormous number of facts on crime, divorce, and abortion rates, but the "causes" are difficult to isolate and weight. Therefore, social scientists will seem to equivocate. In the health field, for example, there is no one definitive explanation for the tremendous increase in expenditures for health services. Thus, policymakers look for scapegoats, rather than looking at the systemic characteristics of health services.

What follows is a list of problems inherent in applied social research. They may also appear in discipline-oriented research. These problems must be coped with as well as possible. They are manageable, given certain working styles, timing, and judgment, much of which is intuitive and difficult to transmit except by example.

1. A constant problem is to find adequate and sympathetic sources of research funding. One must be on the lookout and aggressive. In my case, I happened to be at the right place at

the right time, when funds for health services research were ample.

2. To keep research funds coming, it is necessary to produce results, within a reasonable period, for policy purposes. Action-oriented funding sources expect results to be reasonably within the schedule promised. Be realistic in what you promised.

3. Do not engage in applied research unless such research can be performed with methodology that is already tried and tested. The project must be researchable at that time. This advice is tied in with scheduling.

4. Write two types of reports, if necessary—one for policymakers, and one for your academic peers. It is quite possible to combine them by writing a text that can be understood by the proverbial intelligent layperson. Put detailed tables and explicit methodology in an appendix. In the text, draw on pertinent data, and call attention to the presence of detailed tables in the appendix. Do not make readers interpret your tables: "As seen in Table 4. . . ." Those who want to be critical will consult the tables and the methodology. At the beginning of the report, write an executive summary for the so-called busy policymakers. Obviously, this summary requires a great deal of condensation and confidence in your unqualified data.

5. Much of applied research is interdisciplinary. Such research, contrary to prevailing assumptions that it should be conducted by a team of equals, requires a leader who leads as if there were no leader. Such a leader creates a loose framework of objectives for the research, the methodologies, and the scheduling. The leader needs to have general knowledge of the various skills that go into the methodology, but he or she is a synthesizer. Since applied research is problem- and policy-oriented, the leader must be steeped in knowledge of the policy problems and institutions being researched. It is desirable (although not necessary, since this depends on the personality of the leader) that the leader be older and more experienced than the experts in various methodologies on the research team.

6. Usually, the leader should be the synthesizer of the final report, drawing on the contributions of the members of the

research team. In this case, the leader must be generous in giving credit where credit is due. The team members are climbing the research ladder; the leader is usually already on top, and personal vanity should not interfere with proper allocation of credit. Team members take the bit in their teeth when they know they will be given full credit, and the leader creates a loyalty that cannot be purchased.

7. Finding publishers is never easy. All publishers, even those with sophisticated editorial staffs, send manuscripts to outside reviewers. In a field like health services research, there are many viewpoints on methodology, interpretation, and policy implications. Occasionally, an author gets suggestions for revision, amplification, deletion, or interpretation. All I can say here is to be biased toward yourself; the authors have done more research and thinking on a given research project than any reviewers have done.

8. When a research report has been accepted for publication, cooperate with the editors by quickly returning the edited manuscript and the final galleys. Policy-oriented research ages rapidly. Even the best author or writer needs editing. After living with a project and its write-up for a long time, one becomes bored with rereading and is unable to see defects. My experience with editors has been good. Check for possible errors in interpretation. Do not be "word proud": good editors are trained in the English language, as no scientist has ever been trained. What you need to watch out for is distortion of your style. I have had no trouble in this regard.

9. Whatever your discipline, if you engage in applied social research exclusively (and, to a degree, even in part), you will have to learn how to play a marginal role in the social sciences, between practical research and academia and even within academia.

10. The test of a researcher is the ability to carry through all the stages of a research project—its formulation, implementation, and final product—with constant enthusiasm. The true test is the last stage—carrying through on production after you already know the results. Be as eager to share your results with others as you were to know what the results would be in the

first place. At the same time, do not assume prematurely that you are due for the Nobel Prize.

11. If you become so involved in the severity of social problems and injustice that you are tempted to engage in polemics, then write two reports—one analytical, the other polemical. By *polemics,* I mean outrage with things as they are. This obscures the empirical analysis of what you are outraged about. I probably have the reputation of being too detached, showing no concern. I decided early in my career that I would not burn myself out by feeling outraged, since I did not want to become a cinder too early in my career. My research objectives were for the long-range view.

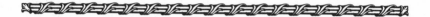

10

A Self-Assessment on Key Contributions

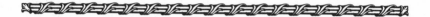

I believe that Nathan Sinai, in the early 1940s, was the first academic to take seriously the development of a health services research unit. Other universities began to follow his example in the 1950s and particularly in the 1960s. The American Sociological Association authorized its Section on Medical Sociology in 1960. I became the section's second chairman in 1961.

I accepted the offer to become director of research at the Health Information Foundation in 1952 because I saw the opportunity to work freely in an independent research foundation with relatively great resources not then available through universities, government, or the mainline philanthropic foundations. The ten years I devoted to the Health Information Foundation, outside a university environment, helped to legitimize health services research as an important area for universities to devote their attention and resources to. In 1952, no university, with the exception of the University of Michigan, seemed to have a serious interest in health services research. It was probably too interdisciplinary. The Health Information Foundation's move to the Graduate School of Business at the University of Chicago, in 1962, provided an interdisciplinary base at that school. Thus, perhaps, one pervasive contribution that I have made is to make health services research a respectable academic mission.

Curiously, it took a sociologist (me) and a public health scholar (Sinai) to open up this area of research. I believe that sociologists' way of conceptualizing was appropriate to the health services enterprise at that time. My major mission was to demonstrate that, in essence, the health services enterprise was a social system, with very few scientifically established performance indicators as to input and output. Hence, the parties at interest are constantly engaged in negotiation and bargaining, in a manner intrinsically different from what obtains in the institutions that produce and sell other kinds of products and services. I find this seemingly self-evident concept difficult to put across to administrators and policymakers, but they still operate as if it is reality. They are always, however, looking for the "holy grail" of certainty.

The nationwide household surveys that I initiated while in New York (and, later, at the University of Chicago) were intended to reveal uses of and expenditures for personal health services on the part of consumers, in order to help define their problems in terms of both public policy and understanding the behavior of the health services system. To change an institution, it seems necessary to understand it first, even partially. Which of its essential characteristics are mutable, and which are resistant by their very nature? These surveys led me into cross-national comparisons, since I discovered that no particular system can be its own reference point. (The U.S.S.R., for example, bought a whole Fiat plant in Italy, moved it to Leningrad, and followed the same mechanical specifications. The only difference was to change the name Fiat to Volga. Health services systems, however, cannot be moved around with such a high degree of specification.)

I also tried to show that part of the basis for disagreement on particular solutions was lack of information, and that perhaps the production of information could reduce disagreement; if not, then one could assume that the disagreement was based on ideology, not on facts. I am partial to the Enlightenment model of social research. Social science is so far (and possibly forever) incapable of emulating the engineering model of the physical sciences (that is, the transferring of physical science's findings to engineers, as is done in engineering schools). The social sciences (even among model-building economists) are incapable of guaranteeing certain results from particular methods. Social science can, however, give us insight into the "nature of the beast," so that administrators and policymakers can be more realistic about the probability of unintended conse-

quences in an enterprise that cannot be controlled, in any sense of
the word. Thus, it is clear why, in pursuing the Enlightenment
model, I selected the survey method and its repetition over time, to
show the dynamics of use and expenditures in the United States. My
cross-national research was based on the same assumption as my
research was on the emergence of HMOs and the promotion of
competition in Minneapolis–St. Paul and Chicago. On an even
more macro scale, this is why I wrote a history of the development
of the health services in the United States from 1875 in terms of the
sociopolitical and economic context that shaped the structure of the
system. I tell my students that they will not learn from me how to
run a health service system, but how to think about it.

In a general sense, I have the impression that my overall
macro research has penetrated the thinking in the field, in both
policy and academia. Still, I have been rather disappointed in the
lack of attention to a systematic study of physicians' decision making on criteria for hospital admission. I also wrote a review article
with Mark Shields (Anderson and Shields, 1982), a physician in an
HMO, in which we were critical of the contemporary conceptualization of quality control and its application to physicians' decision
making. Shields reviewed the clinical literature, and I reviewed the
organizational literature. This was one of the few occasions on
which a physician and a sociologist have collaborated. Shields and
I presented our findings to a meeting jointly sponsored by the major
professional and medical and hospital associations. The theme of
the meeting was quality control. The tenor of the meeting was
upbeat; the need for quality control was in the air. There was un-
critical faith in contemporary methods of quality control, however,
and our presentation was regarded as too pessimistic. We had
scanned the literature thoroughly, but apparently this was not the
time to be critical of an emerging policy to control the profession.
Little reference has been made to this work since then. In due
course, Aspen Publishers offered to publish all the papers delivered
at the meeting. A letter from the health services academic who
helped to organize the meeting, and who was editing the volume,
notified me that our paper would not be included for "lack of
space." I have since come to the conclusion that once the health
policy field gets on the bandwagon of a possible but untested meth-

od of control, criticism is not welcome; the control method has achieved a momentum and vested interests of its own.

In the late 1950s, physicians (and patients) began to be criticized for "overusing" hospitals, as expenditures for hospital care rose rapidly. We had an opportunity to test that allegation operationally in Massachusetts, by taking a sample of hospital discharges and querying the attending physicians about the degree of medical necessity for admitting these patients. For the first time, the field had some operational data on this behavior. We showed that, according to the attending physicians, 11 percent of the surgery, in all likelihood, could have been done outside the hospital. Admissions for 17 percent of the medical patients were also unnecessary, as were 23 percent of the diagnostic admissions. My colleague and I suggested that these percentages revealed the "soft" proportions of hospital admissions, which could be eliminated through proper monitoring. Apparently, however, the medical and administrative practitioners were not ready for such sophisticated systems data, for the study received very little attention.

In summary, I believe that my research contributions to the health services field are largely macrosociological and historical in style. I have tried to introduce conceptual systemic thinking into a field that in itself is a very complex organization. The health services enterprise is a system with boundaries, hierarchies, entry points, and exit points. Administrators and policymakers must accept the fact of unintended consequences and latent functions. There are many "black boxes." The health services problems are illness, suffering, and death. There is a great deal of emotionalism and irrationality. The "customers" are sick and relatively helpless. The healing professional is highly trained and proud and needs a great deal of discretionary authority to function. Health services are constantly problematic. Problems are never resolved—except by the patient's death, when nothing more can be done. Economists, by and large, grossly oversimplify the nature of patients' and physicians' problems, but that is another book.

I have contributed hard and practical data for actuaries, economists, and policymakers about the financial problems of consumers. I have added considerably to the factual universe concerning health services. I have shown that health care is a risk, a contingency, for the individual and the household, by building on the original findings of the Committee on the Costs of Medical Care (1928–1933), on which my mentor, Nathan Sinai, was working. I put CCMC data in up-to-date form in 1954, in a new medical, insurance, and economic context, when private health insurance had become prevalent. I evaluated the impact of this insurance on the consumer. For a decade thereafter, with repeated surveys, I monitored the dynamics of the health services' total national expenditures and the growing effect on consumers of private health insurance. These surveys were widely quoted, and the federal government officially published the results. In time, the federal government took over the periodic surveys, when it became politically comfortable to do so.

I have contributed to the field by opening up the area of cross-national comparisons of health services delivery systems. I showed what the generic problems were in all health services in developed liberal-democratic countries and what the problems were that could be more or less resolved, if not solved.

I have contributed to the understanding of the social, political, and economic environment in which the American health services developed and created the characteristics peculiar to the American "genius" (or "stupidity," as the case may be). Many writers have observed that American history, although a continuation of European, particularly British, history, established different political and social controls and individualistic values; we did not like to emulate European institutions, for they were too close to the Middle Ages and that period's dogmas and hierarchical class system. It is clear that my objectives have been macroanalysis and long-range analysis. I have not attempted to "solve" particular problems; I am a child of the Enlightenment, not of social engineering. The Enlightenment model engages in concepts of society, the human condition, and the values within which institutions evolve. Social engineering puts the technocrat on top—but, worse, the social technocrat is not equal to the engineer in knowledge of physical science. The Enlightenment model is full of awe and humble about the human capacity to control destiny.

Ph.D. students who have been associated with me now have academic positions in thirty universities in this country and a few abroad, and a few are in governmental and other agencies. I have been a guest lecturer at over sixty universities and colleges in this country and abroad.

As for consultants and administrators of hospitals and medical care plans, I estimate I have been associated with over five hundred of them. They are in positions in practically every state in the union and a few foreign countries. The feedback form former students—at conferences, in letters, and through telephone calls—has been generous and heartwarming. My career has been a privilege of the kind accorded to few professors.

What is the future of health services research? What directions will it take? Its future directions will depend on the developments in medical research and their impact on the financing and delivery of health services research and the policies formulated in the political process. In this context, the political process encompasses both public and private initiatives and sources of funding. The increasing emphasis, which has already started, is on a more symmetrical relationship between the patient and the physician, changing the paternalistic charter of the relationship. Inherently, however, this relationship cannot be equal.

Consumers' sovereignty in choice of services will be emphasized. Health services research will continue to be reactive, rather than proactive, because it follows policy and developments, rather than determining policy. This sequence is inherent in the fact that social values evolve in the crucible of human experience. (The Ten Commandments were the result of perhaps five thousand years of human experience, of people learning how to live together in groups and survive as groups.) Research, then, comes along mainly to evaluate the results of experience. Further, research funding can be obtained mainly from public treasuries (taxes) and multimillion-dollar private foundations, both sources with their own agendas, which are not easy to negotiate. Evaluative research deals with actual operations and experiences, not with controlled experiments. The building of abstract models akin to econometric ones will not be funded; even if such models were funded, they would prove too theoretical.

Among policymakers and administrators, the current popu-

larity of health services research is based on the naïve view that facts
will solve problems. They want facts, not theories. Facts can be
supplied. Systemic thinking will take longer, although administrators and policymakers draw on implicit theories of human behavior
and incentives all the time, subconsciously; we could not make
sense of this world as individuals without at least some implicit
theory of human organizational behavior on which we based our
actions, even though much of our theory could be made out to be
nonsense.

The driving force in health services development will be
medical research that can be turned into relatively "quick fixes"
(lasers for cataract operations, pills for ulcer prevention and control
of blood pressure). Organ transplants will become even more sophisticated. The problem will be supply of organ donors, as is
already the case. There will be research on how to motivate people
to be altruistic donors. Medical research in biology and physiology
is at a new frontier, and there will be breakthroughs in genetic
control of diseases that now plague us, such as Parkinson's disease
and epilepsy.

These breakthroughs will worsen our current problems in
bioethics with respect to heroic measures for keeping comatose patients alive. In view of shortages of money and organs, how do we
ration these equitably? Health services research and medical research, as such, cannot resolve these issues. These are moral problems and require fine-tuned philosophical, theological, and legal
discussion that draws on the heritage of these disciplines as applied
to current and unforeseen problems.

Can a working consensus be achieved in our religiously pluralistic society, which ranges from the very orthodox to the atheist?
The most that social research can do is obtain people's attitudes and
beliefs. A new ethic will evolve from human experience. The concept of what is affordable is now being bandied about a great deal.
Implicit in this concept is an ideal health services model that society
can afford and that does not press unduly on desires for other goods
and services—automobiles, vacations, air conditioning, three-bath-
room houses, and all the other amenities that comprise the standard
of living in an affluent society. The concept of affordability is
meaningless, operationally. Continuing medical research will yield

effective and expensive procedures that can justify the spending of 25 to 50 percent of our gross national product, if we value "health" to that extent.

Eventually (and even now, as in Oregon), there will be rationing in closed systems like a government budget or an HMO. Given that eventuality, there may develop a three-level system of basic, intermediate, and wide-open choice, with a price tag for each. There is an illusion that universal health insurance on the Canadian or European model will facilitate an "affordable" health services delivery system for everyone, through payroll deductions and general revenue based on taxes, but no governmental system so far has been able to satisfy all citizens in terms of convenience, choice, amenities, and what is held to be tender loving care. In a liberal-democratic society, the private sector gears up to meet these demands, through private insurance that is parallel or complementary to the public sector's. Then arises the question of equity, which is not settled by research but by dialectics.

Let me list the research projects already in motion, and others still to come, on current perceived and future problems in the health services. They are mainly operational problems, but such problems are still embedded in public and private policy and values. Research can suggest dimensions and alternative approaches with respect to possible costs and potential success.

1. Who are the uninsured, and what will it cost to cover them?
2. Is government getting value for its money by contracting with HMOs for Medicare and Medicaid populations?
3. Are hospitals becoming more efficient through mergers and other methods of operation?
4. What is an adequate supply of health personnel and hospital beds?
5. Is home care more humane and less costly than institutional care? What is a *home*, anyway?
6. Is the concept of diagnostic-related groups (DRGs) working as intended?
7. How workable is the formula, produced by the economist Hsiao at the Harvard School of Public Health, to rationalize physicians' fees specialty by specialty, on the basis of actual

costs of practice and procedures? This is technically known as the resource-based relative value scale (RBRVS).

8. How far can the medical field go into so-called cookbook medicine, relating outcome to diagnosis and treatment in order to make medical practice more "scientific"? The same question can be posed for measurement of quality of services.

9. How effective is competition in containing costs without eroding quality?

10. There will probably be research studying the interface between need or demand and the health services delivery system, to try to rationalize the relationship.

11. The contribution of health services to society will, I hope, be measured by quality of life, rather than length of life.

It seems unlikely that there will be any more nationwide household surveys of use, expenditures, and health insurance of the kind I have been associated with. Syntheses of this kind will no longer be funded. They are not cheap. The U.S. National Center for Health Statistics will probably continue to make sporadic sample surveys of specific data, such as on certain diseases and disabilities. Nevertheless, the excellent annual reports by the Health Care Finance Administration on the financial structure of the United States health services economy will continue. Money will persist as the common denominator for understanding the dynamics of the health services economy, limited as that approach may be.

Cross-national comparisons of health services delivery systems have probably peaked. My research, and that of others, has gone only as far as setting forth the differences and similarities between countries and the more or less commonsense reasons for them, on the basis of precollected data. No further advances can be made in cross-national research without primary research in the "black boxes" of decision making and cultural differences. The logistics of cross-national research are horrendous. Coordination among researchers in various countries is difficult, and I see no funding sources that will come forth with enough money.

Research is unable to suggest to policymakers and administrators what is a possible level of achieving vaguely defined goals. Every social system and every institution limits or liberates, as the case may be, efforts to reach a certain level of achievement. Every goal, even a well-defined one, becomes enmeshed in levels of equilibrium between competing goals and incompatible objectives. This is the human condition. Health services delivery systems are essentially social systems of human relationships, not calibrated machines. Health services research can give some idea, beyond common sense, of the "nature of the beast." Such research is based on the Enlightenment model of knowledge, and not on the social engineering model. "Pushbutton" results cannot be expected in essentially human organizations. The acceptance of this realization can result in more sophisticated and realistic political and administrative negotiating and bargaining methods.

Negotiating and bargaining will be the future of health services delivery systems, mainly because of the lack of scientifically established performance indicators. Such indicators can probably be improved, but the bane of administering the health services will always be the inherent difficulties of relating input to output. Sick customers, and continuing great uncertainty in medical decision making, will be problematic forever.

The proportion of the adult population (not to mention those under eighteen years of age) who will practice a life-style conducive to healthy living—balanced nutrition, exercise, moderate drinking, wearing of seatbelts, and so on—will stabilize at 25 to 35 percent. I make this seat-of-the-pants estimate on the basis of the hedonistic propensities in affluent societies, where consumption patterns have resulted in high rates of morbidity and mortality. Life-style changes have to take place largely as a result of a "religion" of respect for "God's holy vessel," the human body, as illustrated by the Mormons, who eschew tobacco, coffee, and liquor.

This, of course, is the viewpoint of a sociologist. I believe it is fair to say that sociologists opened up the field of health services research in a period of post–World War II affluence, when money, as such, seemed to be no problem. Later, with the cost escalation, economists became dominant in the health services research field.

Resource:
Selected Readings

Aaron, H. J. *Politics and Professors: The Great Society in Perspective*. Washington, D.C.: Brookings Institution, 1978.

Abrams, M. "Political Parties and the Polls." In P. F. Lazarsfeld, W. H. Sewell, and H. L. Wilensky (eds.), *The Uses of Sociology*. New York: Basic Books, 1967.

Andersen, R. M., Aday, L. A., and Fleming, G. V. "A Tale of Two Surveys: Lessons from the Best and Worst of Times in Program Evaluation." In L. Burstein, H. E. Freeman, and P. H. Rossi (eds.), *Collecting Evaluation Data: Problems and Solutions*. Newbury Park, Calif.: Sage, 1985.

Argyris, C. "Creating Effective Relationships in Organizations." *Human Organization*, 1958, *17*, 34-40.

Barber, B. "Research on Research on Human Subjects: Problems of Access to a Powerful Profession." *Social Problems*, 1973, *21*, 103-112.

Beals, R. L. *Politics of Social Research: An Inquiry into the Ethics and Responsibilities of Social Scientists*. Chicago: Aldine, 1969.

Bellah, R. N. "Social Science as Practical Reason." In D. Callahan and B. Jennings (eds.), *Ethics, the Social Sciences, and Policy Analysis*. New York: Plenum Press, 1983.

Berk, R. A., and Rossi, P. H. "Doing Good or Worse: Evaluation Research Politically Examined." *Social Problems*, 1976, *23*, 337-349.

Berns, W., and others. "Is Social Science a God That Failed?" *Public Opinion*, 1981, *4*, 10-15.

Bramson, L. *The Political Context of Sociology.* Princeton, N.J.: Princeton University Press, 1961.

Brauer, C. M. "Kennedy, Johnson, and the War on Poverty." *Journal of American History,* 1982, *69,* 98–119.

Broadhead, R. S., and Rist, R. C. "Gatekeepers and the Social Control of Social Research." *Social Problems,* 1976, *23,* 325–336.

Budrys, G. *Planning for the Nation's Wealth: A Study of Twentieth-Century Developments in the United States.* Westport, Conn.: Greenwood Press, 1986.

Burstein, L., Freeman, H. E., and Rossi, P. H. *Collecting Evaluation Data: Problems and Solutions.* Newbury Park, Calif.: Sage, 1985.

Cain, G. G., and Watts, H. "Problems in Making Policy Inferences from the Coleman Report." *American Sociological Review,* 1970, *35,* 228–242.

Callahan, D., and Jennings, B. *Ethics, the Social Sciences, and Policy Analysis.* New York: Plenum Press, 1983.

Campbell, A., Converse, P. E., and Rodgers, W. L. *The Quality of American Life: Perceptions, Evaluations, and Satisfactions.* New York: Russell Sage Foundation, 1976.

DeSantis, G. "Interviewing as Social Interaction." *Qualitative Sociology,* 1980, *2* (3), 72–97.

Dobson, A., and Bialek, R. "Shaping Public Policy from the Perspective of a Data Builder." *Health Care Financing Review,* 1985, *6* (4), 117–134.

Flook, E. E., and Sanagaro, P. *Health Services Research and R and D in Perspective.* Ann Arbor, Mich.: Health Administration Press, 1973.

Freeman, H. K., Kilcolt, J., and Allen, H. M., II. "Community Health Centers: An Initiative of Enduring Ability." *Milbank Memorial Fund Quarterly/Health and Society,* 1982, *60* (2), 245–267.

Fuller, R. C. "The Problem of Teaching Social Problems." *American Journal of Sociology,* 1938, *44,* 415–425.

Gans, H. J. "Urban Poverty and Social Planning." In P. F. Lazarsfeld, W. H. Sewell, and H. L. Wilensky (eds.), *The Uses of Sociology.* New York: Basic Books, 1967.

Ginzberg, E. "Harder Than It Looks." *Health Services Management Quarterly,* 1989, *11* (2), 19-21.

Glazer, N. *The Limits of Social Policy.* Cambridge, Mass.: Harvard University Press, 1988.

Guillemin, J., and Horowitz, I. L. "Social Research and Political Advocacy." In D. Callahan and B. Jennings (eds.), *Ethics, the Social Sciences, and Policy Analysis.* New York: Plenum Press, 1983.

Habermas, J. *Toward a Rational Society: Student Protest, Science, and Politics.* Boston: Beacon Press, 1970.

Hanft, R. S. "Use of Social Science Data for Policy Analysis and Policy Making." *Milbank Memorial Fund Quarterly/Health and Society,* 1981, *59* (4), 596-613.

Janowitz, M. *Sociology and the Military Establishment.* (Rev. ed.) New York: Russell Sage Foundation, 1965.

Kramer, J. R. "Resistance to Sociological Data: A Case Study." In P. F. Lazarsfeld, W. H. Sewell, and H. L. Wilinsky (eds.), *The Uses of Sociology.* New York: Basic Books, 1967.

Kramer, J. R., and Leventmen, S. *Children of the Gilded Ghetto.* New Haven, Conn.: Yale University Press, 1962.

Lawler, E. E., III, and others. *Doing Research That Is Useful for Theory and Practice.* San Francisco: Jossey-Bass, 1985.

Lippman, W. *A Preface to Politics.* New York: Mitchel Kennedy, 1914.

Lynn, L. E., Jr. (ed.). *Knowledge and Policy: The Uncertain Connection.* Washington, D.C.: National Academy of Sciences, 1978.

McCall, G. J., and Weber, G. H. (eds.). *Social Science and Public Policy: The Role of Academic Disciplines in Policy Analysis.* Port Washington, N.Y.: Associated Faculty Press, 1984.

Maris, P., and Rein, M. *Dilemmas of Social Reform: Poverty and Community Action in the United States.* New York: Atherton Press, 1967.

Martinson, R. "What Works? Questions and Answers About Prison Reform." *Public Interest,* 1974, *35,* 22-34.

Miller, S. M. "The Political Economy of Social Problems, from the Sixties to the Seventies." *Social Problems,* 1976, *24,* 131-141.

Moore, M. H. "Social Science and Policy Analysis: Some Fundamental Differences." In D. Callahan and B. Jennings (eds.),

Ethics, the Social Sciences, and Policy Analysis. New York: Plenum Press, 1983.

Moynihan, D. P. "Policy vs. Program in the '70's." *Public Interest,* Summer 1970, pp. 90-100.

Prewitt, K. "Subverting Policy Premises." In D. Callahan and B. Jennings (eds.), *Ethics, the Social Sciences, and Policy Analysis.* New York: Plenum Press, 1983.

Rein, M. *Social Science and Public Policy.* New York: Penguin Books, 1976.

Reiss, A. J., Jr. "Putting Sociology into Policy." *Social Problems,* 1970, *17,* 289-294.

Reiss, A. J., Jr. "Social and Public Policy." In G. J. McCall and G. H. Weber (eds.), *Social Science and Public Policy: The Role of Academic Disciplines in Policy Analysis.* Port Washington, N.Y.: Associated Faculty Press, 1984.

Rich, R. F. *Social Science Information and Public Policy Making: The Interaction Between Bureaucratic Politics and the Use of Survey Data.* San Francisco: Jossey-Bass, 1981.

Riley, M. W. (ed.). *Sociological Lives: Social Change and Life Course.* Vol. 2. American Sociological Association Presidential Series. Newbury Park, Calif.: Sage, 1988.

Rivlin, A. M. *Systematic Thinking for Social Action.* Washington, D.C.: Brookings Institution, 1971.

Rogers, J. M. *The Impact of Policy Analysis.* Pittsburgh, Pa.: University of Pittsburgh Press, 1988.

Rossi, P. H., and Williams, W. (eds.). *Evaluating Social Programs, Theory, Practice, and Politics.* New York: Seminar Press, 1972.

Sahlins, M. "The Established Order: Do Not Fold, Spindle or Mutilate." In I. L. Horowitz (ed.), *The Rise and Fall of Project Camelot: Studies in the Relationship Between Social Science and Practical Politics.* Cambridge, Mass.: MIT Press, 1967.

Schnaiberg, A. "Obstacles to Environmental Research by Scientists and Technologists: A Social Structural Analysis." *Social Problems,* 1976, *24,* 500-520.

Shotland, R. L., and Marks, M. M. (eds.). *Social Science and Social Policy.* Newbury Park, Calif.: Sage, 1985.

Sinderman, C. J. *Survival Strategies for New Scientists.* New York: Plenum Press, 1987.

Sjoberg, G. (ed.). *Ethics, Politics, and Social Research*. Cambridge, Mass.: Schenkman, 1967.

Sjoberg, G., and Miller, P. J. "Social Research and Bureaucracy." *Social Problems*, 1973, *21*, 129-143.

Smelser, N. J., and Gerstein, D. R. (eds.). *Behavioral and Social Science: Fifty Years of Discovery*. Washington, D.C.: National Academy Press, 1986.

Solovey, M. "John Gillin: From Preacher to Teacher: Religion and Early American Sociology." Unpublished master's thesis, Department of History of Science, University of Wisconsin–Madison, 1988.

Starr, P., and Immergrot, E. "Health Care and the Boundaries of Politics." In C. S. Main (ed.), *Changing Boundaries of the Political: Essays on the Evolving Balance Between the State and Society, Public and Private in Europe*. Cambridge, England: Cambridge University Press, 1987.

Weber, G. H., and McCall, G. J. (eds.). *Social Scientists as Advocates: Views from Applied Disciplines*. Newbury Park, Calif.: Sage, 1978.

Weiss, C. H. *Using Social Research in Public Policy Making*. Lexington, Mass.: Heath, 1977.

Weiss, C. H. "Ideology, Interests, and Information: The Basis of Policy Positions." In D. Callahan and B. Jennings (eds.), *Ethics, the Social Sciences, and Policy Analysis*. New York: Plenum Press, 1983.

Williams, W. "Social Policy Research and Analysis: The Experience of the Federal Social Agencies." New York: Elsevier Science, 1971.

Wilson, W. J. "The Hidden Agenda." *University of Chicago Magazine*, 1987, *80* (1), 4.

References

Aday, L. A., Aitken, M. J., and Wegener, D. H. *Pediatric Care: Results of a National Evaluation of Programs for Ventilator Assisted Children.* CHAS Research Series, no. 36. Chicago: Pluribus Press, 1988.

Aday, L. A., Andersen, R., Loevy, S. S., and Kremer, B. *Hospital-Physician Sponsored Primary Care: Marketing and Impact.* Ann Arbor, Mich.: Health Administration Press, 1985.

Aday, L. A., Fleming, G. V., and Andersen, R. *Access to Medical Care in the United States: Who Has It, Who Doesn't.* CHAS Research Series, no. 32. Chicago: Pluribus Press, 1984.

Andersen, R. *A Behavioral Model of Families' Use of Health Services.* Research Series, no. 25. Chicago: Center for Health Administration Studies, University of Chicago, 1968.

Andersen, R., and Anderson, O. W. *A Decade of Health Services: Social Survey Trends in Use and Expenditures.* Chicago: University of Chicago Press, 1967.

Andersen, R., Lion, J., and Anderson, O. W. *Two Decades of Health Services: Social Survey Trends in Use and Expenditures.* Cambridge, Mass.: Ballinger, 1976.

Andersen, R., Smedby, B., and Anderson, O. W. *Medical Care Use in Sweden and the United States.* Research Series, no. 27. Chicago: Center for Health Administration Studies, University of Chicago, 1970.

Anderson, O. W. *Enabling Legislation for Non-Profit Hospital and Medical Plans.* Research Series, no. 1. Ann Arbor: Bureau of

Public Health Economics, School of Public Health, University of Michigan, 1944.

Anderson, O. W. *Administration of Medical Care: Problems and Issues, Based on an Analysis of the Medical-Dental Care Programs for the Recipients of Old-Age Assistance in the State of Washington, 1941-1945.* Research Series, no. 2. Ann Arbor: Bureau of Public Health Economics, School of Public Health, University of Michigan, 1947.

Anderson, O. W. *Prepayment for Physicians' Services for Recipients of Public Assistance in the State of Washington: Problems and Issues.* Research Series, no. 4. Ann Arbor: Bureau of Public Health Economics, School of Public Health, University of Michigan, 1948.

Anderson, O. W. "The Sociologist in Medicine: Generalizations from a Teaching and Research Experience in a Medical School." *Social Forces,* 1952, *31,* 38-42.

Anderson, O. W. "Age-Specific Mortality Differentials Historically and Currently: Observations and Implications." *Bulletin of the History of Medicine,* 1953a, *27,* 521-529.

Anderson, O. W. "Infant Mortality and Patterns of Living: What Directions Should New Research Take?" *Child,* 1953b, *17,* 122-134.

Anderson, O. W. "Age-Specific Mortality in Selected Western Countries with Particular Emphasis on the Nineteeth Century—Observations and Implications." *Bulletin of the History of Medicine,* 1955, *29,* 3.

Anderson, O. W. "Health Services Systems in the United States and Other Countries: Critical Comparisons." *New England Journal of Medicine,* 1963, *269,* 839-843, 896-900.

Anderson, O. W. *Health Service in a Land of Plenty.* Health Administration Perspective, no. A-7. Chicago: Center for Health Administration Studies, University of Chicago, 1968a.

Anderson, O. W. *The Uneasy Equilibrium: Private and Public Financing of Health Services in the United States, 1875-1965.* New Haven, Conn.: College and University Press, 1968b.

Anderson, O. W. *Health Care: Can There Be Equity? The United States, Sweden, and England.* New York: Wiley, 1972.

Anderson, O. W. *Health Services in the U.S.S.R.* Selected Papers, no. 42. Chicago: Graduate School of Business, University of Chicago, 1973.

Anderson, O. W. *Blue Cross Since 1929: Accountability and the Public Trust.* Cambridge, Mass.: Ballinger, 1975.

Anderson, O. W. *Health Services in the United States: A Growth Enterprise Since 1875.* Ann Arbor, Mich.: Health Administration Press, 1985.

Anderson, O. W. *The Health Services Continuum in Democratic States: An Inquiry into Solvable Problems.* Ann Arbor, Mich.: Health Administration Press, 1989.

Anderson, O. W., Collette, P., and Feldman, J. J. *Changes in Family Medical Care Expenditures and Voluntary Health Insurance: A Five-Year Resurvey.* Cambridge, Mass.: Harvard University Press, 1963.

Anderson, O. W., and Feldman, J. J. *Family Medical Costs and Voluntary Health Insurance: A Nationwide Survey.* New York: McGraw-Hill, 1956.

Anderson, O. W., and May, J. J. *The Federal Employees Health Benefits Program, 1961–1968: A Model for National Health Insurance?* Health Administration Perspective, no. A-9. Chicago: Center for Health Administration Studies, University of Chicago, 1971.

Anderson, O. W., and Sheatsley, P. B. *Comprehensive Medical Insurance: A Study of Costs, Use, and Attitudes Under Two Plans.* Research Series, no. 9. New York: Health Information Foundation, 1959.

Anderson, O. W., and Sheatsley, P. B. *Hospital Use: A Survey of Patient and Physician Decisions.* Research Series, no. 24. Chicago: Center for Health Administration Studies, University of Chicago, 1967.

Anderson, O. W., and Shields, M. "Quality Measurement and Control in Physician Decision Making: State of the Art." *Health Services Research,* 1982, *17,* 125–155.

Anderson, O. W., and others. *HMO Development: Patterns and Prospects: A Comparative Analysis of HMOs.* CHAS Research Series, no. 33. Chicago: Pluribus Press, 1985.

Barber, B. (ed.). *Effective Social Science: Eight Cases in Economics,*

Political Science, and Sociology. New York: Russell Sage Foundation, 1987.

Bellah, R. N. "Social Science as Practical Reason." In D. Callahan and B. Jennings (eds.), *Ethics, the Social Sciences, and Policy Analysis.* New York: Plenum Press, 1983.

Bensman, D. Review of *The Truly Disadvantaged. Dissent,* Spring 1988, pp. 245-246.

Blumer, H. "Social Problems as Collective Behavior." *Social Problems,* 1971, *18,* 299.

Boorstin, D. J. *The Americans: The Democratic Experience.* New York: Random House, 1973.

Bugbee, G. *Reflections of a Good Life: An Autobiography.* Chicago: Hospital Research and Educational Trust, 1987.

Coleman, J. S. Response to receiving the Willard Waller Award from the Section of the Sociology of Education in 1988. *American Sociological Association Footnotes,* 1989, *17* (1), 4.

Coleman, J. S., and others. *Equality of Educational Opportunity.* Washington, D.C.: U.S. Government Printing Office, 1966.

Commons, J. R. *Myself: The Autobiography of John R. Commons.* Madison: University of Wisconsin Press, 1964.

Croog, S. H., and others. "The Effects of Antihypertensive Therapy on the Quality of Life." *New England Journal of Medicine,* 1986, *314,* 1657-1664.

Curti, M., and Carstenson, V. *The University of Wisconsin: A History, 1848 to 1925.* 2 vols. Madison: University of Wisconsin Press, 1949.

Deitchman, S. J. *The Best-Laid Schemes: A Tale of Social Research and Bureaucracy.* Cambridge, Mass.: MIT Press, 1976.

Dickinson, F. "Anderson Versus the U.S. Department of Commerce." *Journal of the American Medical Association,* 1957, *163* (8), 655-656.

Duster, T. Review of *The Truly Disadvantaged. Contemporary Sociology,* 1988, *17* (3), 287.

Editorial. *New England Journal of Medicine,* 1958, *258* (17), 855.

Ely, R. T. *Ground Under Our Feet: An Autobiography.* New York: Macmillan, 1938.

Ewald, W. R., Jr. (ed.). *Environment and Policy: The Next Fifty Years.* Bloomington: Indiana University Press, 1968.

Falk, I. S., Klem, M. C., and Sinai, N. *The Incidence of Illness and the Receipt and Costs of Medical Care Among Representative Families: Experiences in Twelve Consecutive Months During 1928-1931.* Committee on the Costs of Medical Care, publication no. 26. Chicago: University of Chicago Press, 1933.

Feldman, J. J. *The Dissemination of Health Information: A Case Study in Adult Learning.* Chicago: Aldine, 1966.

Fleming, G. V., and Andersen, R. M. *The Municipal Health Services Program: Improving Access While Controlling Costs?* CHAS Research Series, no. 34. Chicago: Pluribus Press, 1986.

Fuller, R. C. "The Problem of Teaching Social Problems." *American Journal of Sociology*, 1938, *44*, 415-425.

Fuller, R. C., and Myers, R. R. "Some Aspects of a Theory of Social Problems." *American Sociological Review*, 1941, *6*, 25.

Gevitz, N. *The D.O.'s: Osteopathic Medicine in America.* Baltimore, Md.: John Hopkins University Press, 1982.

Gibson, G., Bugbee, G., and Anderson, O. W. *Emergency Medical Services in the Chicago Area.* Chicago: Center for Health Administration Studies, University of Chicago, 1971.

Ginzberg, E. "Manpower and Human Resources Policy." In B. Barber (ed.), *Effective Social Science: Eight Cases in Economics, Political Science, and Sociology.* New York: Russell Sage Foundation, 1987.

Ginzberg, E. "Harder Than It Looks." *Health Services Management Quarterly*, 1989, *11* (2), 19-21.

Glazer, N. "The Ideological Uses of Sociology." In P. F. Lazarsfeld, W. H. Sewell, and H. L. Wilensky (eds.), *The Uses of Sociology.* New York: Basic Books, 1967.

Grant, G. "Shaping Policy: The Politics of the Coleman Report." *Teachers College Record*, 1973, *75* (1), 17-54.

Greenlick, M. R., Freeborn, D. K., and Pope, C. R. (eds.). *Health Care Research in an HMO: Two Decades of Discovery.* Baltimore, Md.: John Hopkins University Press, 1988.

Haveman, R. H. *Poverty Policy and Poverty Research: The Great Society and the Social Sciences.* Madison: University of Wisconsin Press, 1987.

Health Information Foundation. Minutes of Executive Committee meeting, New York, Dec. 1, 1952.

Health Information Foundation. Minutes of Executive Committee meeting, New York, Feb. 3, 1953.

Health Information Foundation. Minutes of Board of Directors meeting, New York, May 10, 1957.

Health Information Foundation. "Comprehensive Medical Insurance: A Study of Costs, Use, and Attitudes Under Two Plans." *Progress in Health Services,* 1959, *8* (6).

Hofstadter, R., and Metzger, W. P. *The Development of Academic Freedom in the United States.* New York: Columbia University Press, 1955.

Horowitz, I. L. (ed.) *The Rise and Fall of Project Camelot: Studies in the Relationship Between Social Science and Practical Politics.* Cambridge, Mass.: MIT Press, 1967.

Horowitz, I. L., and Katz, J. E. *Social Science and Public Policy in the United States.* New York: Praeger, 1975.

Janowitz, M. *The Professional Soldier: A Social and Political Portrait.* Glencoe, Ill.: Free Press, 1960.

Janowitz, M. *Sociology and the Military Establishment.* (Rev. ed.) New York: Russell Sage Foundation, 1965.

Janowitz, M. "Military Institutions, the Draft, and the Volunteer Army." In B. Barber (ed.), *Effective Social Science: Eight Cases in Economics, Political Science, and Sociology.* New York: Russell Sage Foundation, 1987.

Jencks, C. Review of *The Truly Disadvantaged. New Republic,* June 13, 1988, p. 32.

Kefauver, E. *In a Few Hands: Monopoly Power in America.* New York: Pantheon Books, 1965.

Kennedy, R. Review of *The Declining Significance of Race. Dissent,* 1979, *26,* 244–247.

Klinghoffer, D. Review of *The Truly Disadvantaged. National Review,* 1988, *40* (4), 47–48.

Law, S. A. *Blue Cross: What Went Wrong?* New Haven, Conn.: Yale University Press, 1974.

Lee, A. M. *Sociology for Whom?* (2d ed.) Syracuse, N.Y.: Syracuse University Press, 1986.

Leggett, J. C. "A Response to Coleman's January 1989 Footnotes." *American Sociological Association Footnotes,* 1989, *17* (5), 7.

Lerner, M. (ed.). *Health Progress in the United States, 1900-1960.* Chicago: University of Chicago Press, 1963.

Lippmann, W. *A Preface to Politics.* New York: Mitchel Kennedy, 1914.

McIntyre, D. M. *Voluntary Health Insurance and Rate Making.* New York: Cornell University Press, 1962.

Martin, R. E. Review of *The Declining Significance of Race. American Political Science Review,* 1980, *74* (2), 523-524.

Mead, L. M. Review of *The Truly Disadvantaged. Commentary,* 1988, *85* (3), 48.

Moynihan, D. P. "Sources of Resistance to the Coleman Report." *Harvard Educational Review,* 1968, *38,* 23-35.

Moynihan, D. P. *Maximum Feasible Misunderstanding: Community Action in the War on Poverty.* New York: Free Press, 1969.

Navarro, V. "Double Standards in the 'Analysis of Marxist Scholarship': A Reply to [A.] Reidy's Critique of My Work." *Social Science and Medicine,* 1985, *20* (5), 441-451.

Nielsen, K. "Emancipatory Social Science and Social Critique." In D. Callahan and B. Jennings (eds.), *Ethics, the Social Sciences, and Policy Analysis.* New York: Plenum Press, 1983.

O'Sullivan, K. "William Julius Wilson: A Bold and Sober Intellect." *American Sociological Association Footnotes,* 1989, *17* (8), 3.

Pettigrew, T. F. Review of *The Declining Significance of Race. Contemporary Sociology,* 1980, *9,* 21.

Pettigrew, T. F., and Green, R. L. "School Desegregation in Large Cities: A Critique of Coleman's 'White Flight' Thesis." *Harvard Educational Review,* 1976, *46* (1), 1-53.

President's Research Committee on Social Trends. *Report on Recent Social Trends in the United States.* New York: McGraw-Hill, 1933.

Rainwater, L., and Yancy, W. L. *The Moynihan Report and the Politics of Controversy.* Cambridge, Mass.: MIT Press, 1967.

Record, W. Review of *The Declining Significance of Race. American Journal of Sociology,* 1980, *85,* 965-968.

Review of *The Truly Disadvantaged. The New Yorker,* Mar. 7, 1988, p. 124.

Ross, E. A. *Social Control: A Survey of the Foundations of Order.* New York: Macmillan, 1924.

Ross, E. A. *Seventy Years of It: An Autobiography.* East Norwalk, Conn.: Appleton-Century-Crofts, 1936.

Runciman, W. G., and Matthews, E., Jr. *Max Weber: Selections in Translation.* Cambridge, England: Cambridge Unversity Press, 1978.

Schulz, R., Girard, C., and Harrison, S. "Management Practices and Priorities for Mental Health System Performance: Evidence from England and West Germany." *International Journal of Health Planning and Management,* 1990, 5 (2), 135-146.

Schuman, H., and Scott, J. "Generations and Collective Memories." American Sociological Review, 1989, *54* (3), 359-381.

Shanas, E. *The Health of Older People: A Special Survey.* Cambridge, Mass.: Harvard University Press, 1962.

Shortell, S. M., and Hughes, E.F.X. "The Effects of Regulation, Competition, and Ownership on Mortality Rates Among Hospital Inpatients." *New England Journal of Medicine,* 1988, *318* (17), 1100-1107.

Shryock, R. H. *The Development of Modern Medicine: An Interpretation of the Social and Scientific Factors Involved.* Madison: University of Wisconsin Press, 1979. (Originally published 1936.)

Sinai, N., and Anderson, O. W. *EMIC: Emergency Maternity and Infant Care: A Study of Administrative Experience.* Research Series, no. 3. Ann Arbor: Bureau of Public Health Economics, School of Public Health, University of Michigan, 1948.

Smiley, J. R., Buck, C. W., Anderson, O. W., and Hobbs, C. E. "Morbidity Experience of Subscribers to a Prepaid Medical Care Plan." *American Journal of Public Health,* 1954, *46,* 367-371.

Streeten, P. (ed.). *Gunnar Myrdahl: Value in Social Theory: A Selection of Essays on Methodology.* New York: Harper & Row, 1958.

Sydenstricker, E. *Health and Environment.* New York: McGraw-Hill, 1933.

U.S. Bureau of the Census. *U.S. Census of Manufacturers: 1958.* Vol. 2: *Industry Statistics, Part I. Major Groups 20 to 28.* C.P.A. no. 96. Washington, D.C.: U.S. Bureau of the Census, 1961.

U.S. Congress, House of Representatives. *Behavioral Sciences and the National Security.* Part IX: *Winning the Cold War: The U.S. Ideological Offensive, July 8, 13, and 14 and August 4, 1965.* 89th Congress, 2nd session. Washington, D.C.: U.S. Government Printing Office, 1965.

U.S. Congress, House of Representatives. *Behavioral Sciences and the National Security.* House Report no. 1224. Washington, D.C.: U.S. Government Printing Office, 1966.

Waitzkin, H. "Truth's Search for Power: The Dilemmas of Social Sciences." *Social Problems,* 1968, *15,* 408–419.

Weinberg, J. *Edward Alsworth Ross and the Sociology of Progressivism.* Madison: State Historical Society of Wisconsin, 1972.

Wilson, W. J. *The Declining Significance of Race: Blacks and Changing American Institutions.* Chicago: University of Chicago Press, 1978.

Wilson, W. J. "The Hidden Agenda." *University of Chicago Magazine,* 1987a, *80* (1), 4.

Wilson, W. J. *The Truly Disadvantaged: The Inner City, the Underclass, and Public Policy.* Chicago: University of Chicago Press, 1987b.

Index